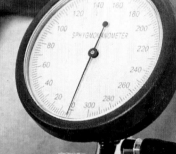

The Essential Guide to
Blood Pressure

SERIES EDITOR

NEWHAM LIBRARIES

9080101097560

Published in Great Britain in 2019 by
need2know
Remus House
Coltsfoot Drive
Peterborough
PE2 9BF
Telephone 01733 898103
www.need2knowbooks.co.uk

All Rights Reserved
© Need2Know
SB ISBN 978-1-91084-396-3
Cover photograph: Adobe Stock

Contents

Chapter 5: How Hypertension Affects You 47

Chapter 6: Low Blood Pressure: Causes and Treatment 57

Chapter 7: Lifestyle Changes to Treat Hypertension 67

Chapter 8: Treatments for Hypertension 77

Chapter 9: Dealing with the Treatment Pros and Cons 89

Introduction

This book is a useful read for anyone wishing to understand their blood pressure. Few of us fully understand what blood pressure is or why it's such a big deal, though we hear about it all the time. Pressures on your doctors' time means that they can't always answer all of your questions. This book should be like having your own personal doctor with all the time in the world to answer your questions on blood pressure.

"High blood pressure" is one of the most common topics we'll hear on the subject. High blood pressure affects more than 1 in 4 adults in England, and medications to keep this under control are taken by millions of people. Low blood pressure can also occur, though this is far less common.

The Essential Guide to Blood Pressure aims to explain clearly how blood pressure can be abnormal, and what the term "blood pressure" actually means. It is based on research by qualified medical professionals who have spent years researching hypertension and working with patients living with high blood pressure. This research comes from people with first-hand understanding of all there is to know about blood pressure and hypertension.

It's common to wish you had more time to discuss the details of your condition with your doctor, but sadly this isn't always possible. Many people end up walking out of their appointments with medication for a condition they don't fully understand. Our goal with this book is to help you have a better understanding of what the treatment is for. This information, combined with lifestyle advice and discussions of alternative blood pressure remedies should mean that by the end of the book you will have enough information to put your own blood pressure plan into action.

Rigorously conducted scientific studies are the source for all of the information in this book, and we have tried to include all of the latest evidence at the time of printing.

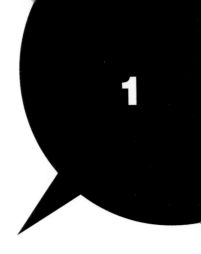

1

Blood Pressure

Your Circulation

The blood circulating around your body acts as a transport system – it supplies your cells with the glucose and oxygen that they need to make energy and it takes their waste products away.

The organs in your body are made up of millions of different cells, all working together. Your kidneys, heart, stomach and brain are all classed as organs, and are made from groups of cells that function similarly. These cells need to be able to get rid of any waste products that build up inside them in order to function properly, and they need access to energy.

Arteries

The majority of your arteries carry blood that is rich in oxygen from the left side of your heart and distributes this to all the cells in your body.

- The blood vessels that take blood away from the heart are known as arteries

- Oxygen-rich blood is carried by the arteries

- Arteries carry blood to other organs in your body

Although most arteries carry blood that contains high levels of oxygen, there are some arteries that transport blood which is low in oxygen. These are known as "pulmonary arteries". They're responsible for carrying blood from your heart to your lungs, where they can increase its oxygen levels.

In order to reach all of your cells, the arteries furthest from your heart are very small. The artery that leaves the heart, known as the "aorta", is very large.

Your Veins

- The blood vessels that take blood away from other organs are known as veins

- Blood that is low in oxygen is usually carried by the veins

- Veins bring blood back to your heart

Your veins carry your blood back to the heart after your cells have taken all the glucose and oxygen that they need from it. This means blood in veins generally contains far less oxygen than the blood in your arteries. The "pulmonary vein" is the only vein that carries blood rich in oxygen. This vein brings blood from the lungs to the heart, after it's been topped up with oxygen.

The Heart

- The heart is made from powerful muscles that pump blood all around the body

- Your heart beats on average 70-80 times per minute

- Your heart doesn't just beat at a constant rate throughout your life; it can vary depending on what you are doing

- It has to pump blood up to your brain as well as down to your big toe!

The heart is essentially a big pump made out of muscle. It's divided into two sides: left and right. Blood from the veins enters the right side of the heart, which pumps it to the lungs so that it can pick up oxygen. This blood then flows to the left side of the heart, which pumps it to the rest of your organs.

"It is often said that members of royal families have blue blood, but the colour of your blood has nothing to do with whether you are royalty. Blue blood just contains less oxygen than bright red blood."

Your heart will beat all day, every day, for as long as you live. It has to be the strongest muscle in your body, as it's responsible for keeping you alive.

When you go for a run the cells in your leg muscles have to work very hard and need a lot more energy. In order for them to get all the oxygen-rich blood they need, the heart has to beat much faster than usual.

When you're asleep, your cells don't need to work as hard as they do when you're up and about. This means your heart can slow down for a while, as your cells produce less waste and require less energy, so they don't need your heart to pump so much blood.

Your Blood Pressure

- The pressure of the blood in your arteries is referred to as "blood pressure"
- "Millimetres of mercury" is the measurement used to record blood pressure
- Your blood pressure has two components
- "Systolic" blood pressure is recorded in the upper number of your blood pressure
- The lower number is the "diastolic" blood pressure
- The pressure of blood in your veins is not a part of your blood pressure reading

"It is estimated that your heart will beat more than 2 billion times in your lifetime."

In a central heating system, the amount of pressure needed to force water through pipes will depend on the size of the pipes. The smaller the diameter of a pipe, the greater the pressure required. The pump in your central heating system will work at a constant pressure to keep water flowing through your pipes.

When doctors measure pressure in your arteries they use the units 'millimetres of mercury' (mmHg). Just like centimetres is a standard way of talking about distance, this is the standard way to discuss pressure. The stiffness of the walls of your arteries and the blood your heart pumps into them creates the pressure in your arteries. The pressure needed to force blood through the arteries will be increased if they are narrow and stiff.

The pressure system in your body is more dynamic than that of a central heating system, so it's a little more complicated. The rate and force of your heart's pumping ability can be altered by nerves that supply your heart. Meanwhile, the diameter of your blood vessels can be altered by the nerves that supply them. This means your blood pressure can be adjusted by your body depending on its needs at the time. Whatever you're up to, your blood pressure can be adjusted to suit.

When your blood pressure is recorded, it'll be presented as a fraction:

$$\frac{\text{upper blood pressure}}{\text{lower blood pressure}}$$

What the Upper Number Means: Systolic Blood Pressure

Just like when you switch your central heating system on the pump will increase the pressure in your water pipes, the pressure within your arteries is increased when your heart pumps blood into them.

The pressure in your arteries will generally increase to around 120mmHg when your heart pumps. This is the upper blood pressure number that your doctor will give you, known as the **systolic blood pressure**.

Every time your heart pumps the pressure in your arteries increases to around 120mmHg and then falls again as your heart relaxes. There is no "constant level" when it comes to blood pressure. Throughout your circulation, the pressure generated when your heart pumps will pulsate approximately 80 times per minute. When you take your pulse, this is what you can feel.

Diastolic Blood Pressure – What the Lower Number Means

The lower pressure in your arteries is called the diastolic blood pressure and is usually around 70mmHg. Your heart has to relax and get ready for the next beat after each time it pumps blood into your arteries. Blood still needs to flow to your cells when your heart relaxes, however, so it never drops to zero.

The arteries contain blood at all times, and the walls of the arteries have muscle tone, so they're able to create a pressure of their own. This is how the diastolic blood pressure is maintained.

What Is "Normal"?

"Normal" blood pressure is the widely accepted goal for blood pressure tests. It's taken many years of scientific study to figure out what normal blood pressure is, so it's worth thinking about it!

How Do Doctors Know what a Normal Blood Pressure Is?

Charting "Normal"

To calculate this range, over many years scientists have taken the blood pressure of thousands of healthy people.

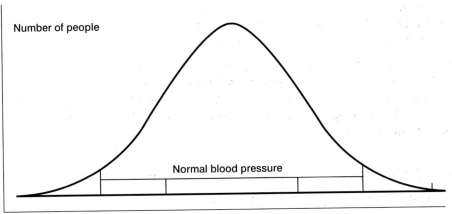

"A perfectly normal person is rare in our civilization."
Karen Horney, German Psychoanalyst.

People can have a wide range of different blood pressures, just like they can be various heights and have various skin colours. This means there's a range of both diastolic and systolic blood pressures that are classed as normal, rather than a single blood pressure measurement.

The "normal" or "bell shaped" curve is taken by plotting the blood pressure readings of thousands of healthy people onto a graph. The "normal" part of the curve is the range in the middle of the graph, where most people's blood pressure will lie.

The Association between Blood Pressure and Disease

The main illnesses that high blood pressure causes are heart attacks, angina and strokes. Although the people originally used to create this "normal range" were healthy at the time of testing, they may have developed problems due to their blood pressure later in life. This makes the idea of normal blood pressure a little more complicated than just plotting it on a graph.

To deal with this complication, doctors have taken blood pressure readings from thousands of "healthy" people, and followed them up over time to see if their blood pressure has caused them to develop any problems later on. The blood pressure measurements deemed less likely to cause illness in later life are the ones that have been classed as "normal".

So What Is Normal?

- Systolic blood pressure between 90 and 130mmHg is classed as normal
- A normal diastolic blood pressure is between 60 and 85mmHg

Do My Veins also Have a Blood Pressure?

The blood pressure in your veins is much lower – usually around 5 to 7mmHg. One way valves are needed to stop your blood from flowing backwards in veins.

Your arteries are used to provide the type of blood pressure readings that your doctor will give you.

Your muscles and other organs exert pressure on your veins, and this is the main force that drives blood back to the heart through the veins.

Blood Pressure at Different Ages

The pressure in your arteries will change throughout your life, as well as on a minute to minute basis.

Blood Pressure in the Growing Child

At birth, a baby's blood pressure is between 65-95/30-60. Adults have higher blood pressure than young children and infants. Blood pressure tends to reach adult values at around 18 years old, having gradually increased throughout childhood.

Pregnancy and Blood Pressure

The heart doesn't have to pump as forcefully to drive blood through the arteries during a healthy, regular pregnancy, as the hormone progesterone causes the arteries to relax. This means it's common to have a lower blood pressure than normal during pregnancy.

Should My Blood Pressure Increase as I Get Older?

As they age, the blood pressure of people in the western world tends to increase. This increase in blood pressure throughout life is what causes high amounts of blood pressure related disease in western society. This was believed to be normal at one time.

But when scientists studied the blood pressure of tribal societies who lived active, hunter-gatherer lifestyles, it was found that even in those around 70 years old there was no increase in blood pressure. These societies also weren't affected by the same blood pressure related diseases that we in the western world have to worry about.

We now believe that a poor diet containing too much salt and an inactive lifestyle are contributing to Westerners' rise in blood pressure with age.

Summing Up

- Your heart pumps blood through your arteries, and this is what causes blood pressure.

- Your blood pressure should not be increasing as you age.

- The residual pressure in your arteries when your heart muscle is relaxed is measured to give the lower number (diastolic blood pressure).

- The upper number (systolic blood pressure) reflects the pumping force of your heart.

- Blood pressure is low in children and pregnant women, but for the rest of your life your blood pressure should be between 90-139/60-89mmHg.

2

Blood Pressure Tests

How Is Blood Pressure Measured?

The method of blood pressure is standard all over the world. The pressure in your arteries rapidly rises to the systolic blood pressure each time your heart beats, before falling back down to the diastolic. This means that if your blood pressure measures 120/80, the pressure in your arteries will begin at 80mmHg before suddenly jumping to 120mmHg every time your heart beats – around 80 times every 60 seconds.

Blood pressure is usually measured on your arm, just above the elbow. Your doctor will need to detect both the lower and upper values of this pressure pulsation in order to measure your blood pressure. A "Sphygmomanometer" – a manometer, a piece of equipment used to measure pressure, attached to an inflatable cuff – is used to measure this.

The brachial artery is generally used to measure your blood pressure – it is accessible, running close to the skin on your arm.

As long as the equipment used the same, your blood pressure measurement should be the same in the UK as it is in the US, as the measurement is an international standard.

Systolic (Upper) Blood Pressure

The doctor will place a cuff around your upper arm, which will then be inflated to a pressure level greater than your systolic blood pressure level. This will cut off blood flow to your arm through the brachial artery. The doctor will then slowly reduce the pressure in the cuff until it is the same as your systolic level. By listening just above or below your elbow with a stethoscope, the doctor will be able to hear when the levels are the same as the blood will start flowing through the artery again, creating a pulsation which they will hear as a tapping sound.

The upper number – your systolic blood pressure – is the pressure at which the doctor can start to hear this pulsation.

Measuring the Diastolic Blood Pressure

Having recorded your systolic number, the doctor will deflate the cuff further so that the pressure falls just below diastolic pressure. When they reach this point, the blood in the artery will no longer be audible through the stethoscope. The lower number – your diastolic blood pressure – is the pressure just before the pulsing becomes inaudible.

Blood Pressure Machines

In the past, machines used to measure blood pressure had a mercury manometer and a cuff that had to be pumped up by hand. Other manometers have since been brought in to replace this design, as mercury can be harmful. Many newer blood pressure machines are still compared against the older design as it was very accurate and produced the gold standard of blood pressure measurement.

This means that blood pressure readings taken by your doctor, in the old fashioned way, can be compared to those taken by electronic meters.

Electronic or Digital Machines

The newest machines used to measure blood pressure are electronic, rather than manual. Some of these machines can also store blood pressure readings so there is a record of how your blood pressure changes over time. Stethoscopes are no longer needed as there's equipment inside the cuff that can detect sounds, and the cuff is inflated automatically rather than with a pump.

Electronic Machine Standardisation

The blood pressure readings you get from different electronic blood pressure machines can differ because there are many different makes on the market which are all slightly different in design. So, your blood pressure could be very different on one machine compared to another. This is the main problem with the modernised system.

The old fashioned sphygmomanometer is used as a point of comparison for some electronic blood pressure monitors to ensure that the readings are as accurate and consistent as possible. Rigorous testing is necessary to make sure this is the case.

Doctors will only take your blood pressure with the properly tested and reliable meters, as some electronic meters are more reliable than others. It is important that your doctor know for certain that any changes in readings are not because of a change in machines but a change in your health.

Measuring Blood Pressure at Home

Why Is It Necessary?

- You'll get a better sense of what your blood pressure is normally like if you measure it at home.

- Finding out how your blood pressure varies throughout the day can be interesting.

- Patients who take their own blood pressure have better blood pressure control.

- It will get you involved in your own care.

Which Machine Should I Buy?

- Whatever your reason for buying a machine, when you go into a shop or look online you will be faced with a plethora of machines and choosing can be difficult.

- There are so many different blood pressure machines out there.

- Some machines have been tested more rigorously than others and are more reliable.

- Your doctor should be able to recommend a good one.

- The prices of machines can vary considerably.

- It can be a false economy to buy a machine just because it is cheap.

- Machines that measure blood pressure using a cuff placed around the upper arm are, at the moment, usually more reliable than finger or wrist blood pressure monitors.

"Many people want to measure their own blood pressure. This is usually because they find that their blood pressure at home is much lower than when they are stressed in the GP surgery."

No matter how relaxing, reassuring and informal your doctor tries to be, sitting in a room with someone who knows more about your health than you do can be an understandably worrying experience – enough to put anyone's blood pressure up! Measuring your own blood pressure is a good option for many people. You may well find that you'll get a better idea of what your blood pressure is really like if you take blood pressure readings at home.

A lot of people buy a blood pressure machine out of academic interest because they want to see how their blood pressure changes over the course of the day.

Which Machine Is Best?

You'll need to use a stethoscope with some home blood pressure monitors as they work like the old fashioned ones. However, people will usually opt for an electronic machine as they find the old fashioned version difficult to use. If you want to compare your blood pressure readings with those of your doctor it is better if you buy a machine that is known to produce similar readings to the one used by your doctor.

If you are just buying a machine to see how your blood pressure varies and are only going to be comparing the results with those from the same machine then the type of machine you buy is less important.

Unless your doctor can suggest one that is reliable, it's currently the best idea to avoid wrist and finger monitors as they don't tend to work as well as monitors with upper arm cuffs. This still leaves loads of different kinds of arm blood pressure monitors to choose from though, so don't worry!

There Are So Many Machines on the Market, Is There a Way to Choose?

Your budget and your reasons for buying a blood pressure monitor will determine the best machine for you. Your GP should be happy to tell you which type they use, and what similar models are available.

The British Hypertension Society website (**www.bhsoc.org**) has an up-to-date list of recommended machines and their prices. This list is updated regularly as new machines are being developed all the time.

What Do I Need to Consider?

The cuff should fit snugly around your arm, it shouldn't easily slip off and it shouldn't be too tight. If the cuff doesn't fit you properly the blood pressure readings will be wrong. The size of the cuff on your machine will be very important. If you're unsure which cuff size you should get, ask your doctor or nurse.

- The standard size cuff that comes with the monitor will be fine for most people.

- You may need to get a larger cuff if you find it difficult to do up the standard cuff.

- If your arms are thin and the cuff slips down your arm easily, you will need to get a smaller cuff.

How Should I Measure My Blood Pressure at Home?

Before you start taking any readings make sure that you know how to work the machine. Rest for a couple of minutes beforehand and try not to talk while you are doing it. You should be sitting down with your legs uncrossed when you take your blood pressure, unless your doctor has told you otherwise.

The crease in your elbow should be around 2cm below the cuff. While the machine is working, you should rest your arm on a desk or table at the level of your heart.

Only start recording your measurements when you are happy using the machine, otherwise stress associated with not knowing how to use the machine will put your blood pressure up. Don't write your measurements down the first few times you try using the machine. Sometimes the machines will take a while or make a couple of attempts; don't worry if this happens – just be patient.

How to Measure Your Blood Pressure

1   Rest for a few minutes while sitting down.

2   Try not to talk or cross your legs.

3   Rest your arm on a table at the level of your heart (just below your nipple).

4   Wrap the cuff around your arm, slightly above the elbow.

5   When it's not inflated, the cuff should fit snugly around the arm.

6   Try not to move while the machine is working.

Perhaps someone could help put the cuff on your arm, or write down the readings for you. When you're using the blood pressure machine at home, it's a good idea to get someone in your family to help you figure it out. This will help your family to feel involved, as well as making the process of putting on the cuff and working the machines less challenging overall.

When Should I Measure My Blood Pressure at Home?

It's a good idea to take your blood pressure a couple of times throughout the day. Stick to these times (half an hour either side should make no difference) and record your blood pressure for a few days. For instance, you could measure it at breakfast time, lunchtime and just before bed.

If you're on holiday your blood pressure may be much lower than it is at the office, which will give you great readings, but not ones that are representative of your true blood pressure for most of your life. When you're recording your blood pressure, try to capture your everyday life.

It's best to avoid coffee or energy drinks for around 30 minutes before you plan to test your blood pressure, as caffeine can put your blood pressure up. Don't forget to write both the systolic and diastolic readings down so both you and your doctor can see what is happening to your blood pressure over time.

How Often Should I Measure It?

Try to choose certain times on certain days to check your blood pressure and try not to check in between times. Many people will become so worried about their blood pressure that they take hundreds of readings in the hope that they will eventually be normal. Don't develop an obsession, but it is important that you measure your blood pressure regularly if you're doing it for medical reasons.

Your blood pressure readings may appear worse than they really are if you're thinking too much about them, as it can become difficult to relax.

Ask your doctor or nurse if you aren't sure how often and what times will work best for you.

My Doctor Thinks I May Have White Coat Hypertension, What Is This?

Visiting the doctor can be a stressful experience for many people. You have to think about traffic and timing and getting off work in order to get there on time. And there always seem to be more patients than parking spaces, so parking at the surgery can seem impossible. All of these things can affect your blood pressure, so it's not unusual to have higher blood pressure at the doctor's office than at home. "White coat hypertension" is the term given to this issue.

When they are away from the surgery, some people with white coat hypertension will have perfectly normal blood pressure which just goes up when they get to the GP. Some will have high blood pressure at all times, but it will be even higher when they get to the surgery.

Checking your blood pressure at home is a good idea if you believe you could have white coat hypertension. If you buy your own machine for this purpose make sure it is one of the recommended and reliable ones. This will also get you involved with your own health, which can only be a good thing.

I Think I Have White Coat Hypertension

Mention it to your doctor if you think that you could have white coat hypertension. They may well agree with you, and can give you a blood pressure machine that will allow you to measure your own blood pressure from home.

Twenty-Four Hour Blood Pressure Monitoring Explained

Ambulatory blood pressure monitoring is another name given to twenty-four hour blood pressure monitoring.

What Has to Be Done?

You'll have to wear a machine that monitors your blood pressure for 24 hours if it's recommended that you try ambulatory blood pressure monitoring. This will involve wearing a small monitor around your waist, attached to a cuff placed around your upper arm. It should not interfere with your normal daily life as the equipment is small and discreet.

At regular intervals, the cuff will inflate itself – this is usually every half hour at night and every 15 minutes during the day. Before it inflates, it will generally beep so that you can sit down and rest your arm ahead of testing. Try to keep your arm still when the machine is working, but don't worry if you aren't always able to sit down.

Your sleep may be disturbed by the inflation of the blood pressure cuff during a 24 hour recording. When your doctor is interpreting the readings they may want to take this into account, so don't be afraid to tell them if the machine has kept you awake.

"Sometimes your doctor may just ask you to wear the equipment for 12 rather than 24 hours."

Why Do I Need a 24-Hour Blood Pressure Recording?

Your doctor will be able to see exactly what your blood pressure is doing over the whole day if you have a 24-hour record of it.

Your doctor may request a 24-hour blood pressure recording…

- because they are unsure whether or not to treat your blood pressure when it's slightly higher than usual;
- if they want to see how your blood pressure is outside of the doctor's surgery;
- to see how your blood pressure varies throughout the day;
- to see if your treatment is working.

Summing Up

- A variety of machines can be used to measure blood pressure.

- When measuring blood pressure, the most important thing is that the reading is reliable and precise. It should be taken on a machine that can be compared safely to other machines, having been rigorously tested and approved.

- You may be asked to wear a 24 hour blood pressure monitor or check your own blood pressure at home if your doctor needs more information than a one-off reading can give.

- If possible whenever your blood pressure is being taken you should sit down with your legs uncrossed and your arm resting on a table at the height of your heart.

- Some machines are more reliable than others, in particular, at the present time, most machines that measure blood pressure in your wrist or finger are not as good as ones that measure blood pressure in your upper arm.

- The machines can be manual or electronic, but most patients find it easier to use electronic machines.

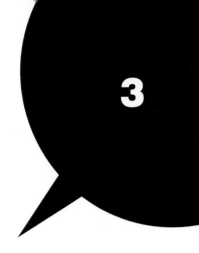

3

Understanding Hypertension

The numbers quoted in this book are from the British Hypertension Society; an organisation that produces guidelines for the UK. Different countries tend to have slightly different ideas of normal blood pressure and different treatment recommendations. This means it can be a little confusing to read about the classification of blood pressure on the Internet.

The general concepts and levels of blood pressure that require treatment are the same in most countries, even though the guidelines available in different countries may be slightly different to those included in this book.

High Blood Pressure

If either the diastolic (lower) or systolic (upper) numbers – or both – are elevated, your blood pressure may be abnormally high.

- The term "isolated systolic hypertension" is used if only the systolic number is high.
- The word "hypertension" is used on its own if both numbers are elevated.
- If only the lower number is elevated this is called "isolated diastolic hypertension".

Your risk of dying from a stroke or heart attack doubles with every 20mmHg your blood pressure increases.

Treatment Isn't Always Necessary (The Grey Areas)

"Doctors refer to high blood pressure as 'hypertension'. 'Hyper' means high and 'tension' means pressure.

- Blood pressure with a lower reading below 85mmHg and an upper reading above 130mmHg is classed as normal.

So I Am Not at Risk from My Blood Pressure if It Is Below 130/85mmHg?

We now understand that the risks associated with having high blood pressure begin to increase once the blood pressure rises above 115/75. The risks are not great enough at this stage to warrant treatment, however, so doctors do not offer treatment for blood pressure of this level.

High Normal

"Pre-hypertension" and "high normal" are phrases now used to describe blood pressures that fall between 130/85 and 139/89. The risks existing within this range need to be weighed up against the side effects, costs and risks that come with treatment itself, but it should be kept in mind that readings around this level have been linked with a higher risk of stroke and heart attack. As a general rule, treatment isn't offered to people with pre-hypertension.

If you have pre-hypertension, your doctor will ask you to come for annual check-ups and will want to keep a close eye on your blood pressure, as many people with pre-hypertension go on to develop true hypertension and will require treatment.

When Does High Blood Pressure Require Treatment?

In America, high blood pressure killed over 55,000 people in 2005 alone, according to the American Heart Association. It's believed that a third of adults have high blood pressure.

You can be diagnosed with hypertension in three ways:

- Your GP has determined your blood pressure to be high on at least 3 separate visits.
- Your blood pressure is found to be high on a 24-hour blood pressure monitor.
- If your home blood pressure readings taken on a reliable machine are consistently high.

Mild High Blood Pressure

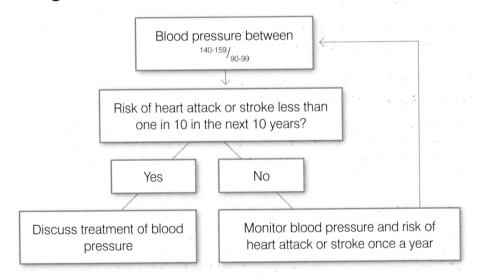

"Doctors divide high blood pressure into three main categories; mild, moderate and severe hypertension."

Blood pressure between 140/90 and 159/99 is classed as mild hypertension. Your doctor will start to think about giving you treatment if your blood pressure reaches this range.

Your other risk factors for suffering from strokes, heart attacks or angina later in life will determine whether or not you need treatment at this point. If your risk is low (usually said to be less than a 1 in 10 (or 10%) chance of suffering a heart attack or stroke in the next 10 years) your doctor will continue to check your blood pressure and risk every year, but will not offer you treatment.

High blood pressure is a significant contributor to this risk – the risk of suffering from these conditions is known as "cardiovascular risk".

If your risk increases to more than a 10% chance of suffering a stroke or heart attack in the next 10 years, or your blood pressure rises above 160/99mmHg, your doctor will advise treatment.

I Suffer from Diabetes, Does That Make Any Difference?

Your risk of having a stroke or heart attack is increased if you have diabetes when compared to the risk of those who don't have the condition. This means that regardless of your calculated cardiovascular risk, it's recommended that you start treatment for your blood pressure if it rises above 140/90.

Calculating Cardiovascular Risk

Your likelihood of developing angina, stroke or heart attack is known as cardiovascular risk. There are various different equations that doctors use to calculate this risk. In most cases, this is calculated as a percentage risk of suffering from these conditions in the next decade. You can find some of the equations online, such as…

- Framingham Risk Score
- Absolute Risk Calculator
- The ASSIGN score (tailored to a Scottish population)

What Factors Are Used in these Equations?

- Upper blood pressure
- Whether you're a smoker or non-smoker
- Your biological sex
- Your age
- Your cholesterol

Certain equations also take into consideration whether your blood pressure will have already damaged your heart, and whether or not you have diabetes.

Moderate to Severe Hypertension

- A blood pressure above 180/110 is classed as severe hypertension.
- Moderate hypertension is defined as blood pressure over 160/100.

Regardless of your cardiovascular risk, your doctor will advise that you receive treatment for moderate to severe hypertension.

	Systolic Blood Pressure (mmHg)	Diastolic Blood Pressure (mmHg)
Severe Hypertension	Greater than 180	Greater than 110
Moderate Hypertension	160-179	100-109
Mild Hypertension	140-159	90-99
Pre-Hypertension	130-139	85-89
Normal blood pressure	Less than 130	Less than 85

Isolated Systolic Hypertension

What Does It Mean?

You have isolated systolic hypertension if your upper number (systolic blood pressure) is consistently higher than 140mmHg but the lower number is below 90mmHg.

- Isolated systolic hypertension is associated with a high cardiovascular risk.
- Isolated systolic hypertension is defined as a blood pressure of >140/<90mmHg.

Is Isolated Systolic Hypertension Important?

Systolic blood pressure was once believed to be an inevitable consequence of ageing due to a hardening of the arteries. As a result, doctors believed that it wasn't a big deal.

"Large studies that have measured thousands of people's blood pressure and then observed what happens to these people in future years have found that systolic blood pressure is actually more important than diastolic blood pressure."

At this time, doctors thought that diastolic blood pressure was the most important reading, and that systolic blood pressure didn't make a major difference. However, people with systolic blood pressure are far less likely to suffer from future angina, strokes or heart attacks than those whose systolic blood pressure is raised.

Higher Diastolic Blood Pressure

What Is Isolated Diastolic Hypertension?

You have isolated diastolic hypertension if your lower (diastolic) blood pressure reading is higher than 90mmHg while your systolic blood pressure is normal.

- Isolated diastolic hypertension is less common than isolated systolic hypertension.
- Isolated diastolic hypertension is defined as a blood pressure of <140/>90mmHg.

Is It a Big Deal?

If you are younger than 50 years old having high diastolic blood pressure puts you at a greater risk of suffering from a heart attack, angina or stroke. Your age will determine whether or not isolated diastolic hypertension is a big issue. Many doctors believe that isolated diastolic hypertension isn't important if you're over 50 years old.

High Blood Pressure during Pregnancy

Your cardiovascular system will normally adjust to provide enough blood supply to the placenta and developing foetus during pregnancy. Due to the effects of the hormone progesterone, one of the adjustments your body makes is that blood pressure will fall slightly during the second trimester (after 12 weeks).

If you do develop high blood pressure when you're pregnant, it could have a negative impact for both you and the baby. The main problem of having high blood pressure during pregnancy is that it can limit the amount of blood getting through the placenta to the growing embryo. This can make it difficult for the baby to grow properly, as they won't be getting all the nutrients and oxygen they need.

However, if your blood pressure is only slightly elevated, it shouldn't be a problem and your doctor will just want to keep an eye on it to make sure it doesn't increase further.

Hypertension during Pregnancy – Some Definitions

Chronic Hypertension

This tends to last more than three months after delivery, having started before the 20th week of pregnancy. The only difference between this and regular hypertension is that it just happens to have developed during pregnancy.

Pregnancy Induced Hypertension (PIH)

Also known as gestational hypertension, this develops after the 20 week mark and goes away once you've given birth. Women who suffer from gestational hypertension are more likely to have high blood pressure later in life, though pregnancy is the cause of gestational hypertension itself.

Pre-Eclampsia

Pre-eclampsia can be mild, moderate or severe; if it is mild the doctors will keep an eye on it. After 20 weeks of pregnancy, you can be diagnosed with pre-eclampsia if you have high blood pressure and protein is found in your urine. Although doctors monitor women's blood pressure during pregnancy and will check the urine for any protein if the blood pressure is raised, pre-eclampsia can also come on suddenly.

This can be a serious condition for both you and your baby if it's in its severe form. You should contact your doctor immediately if you are pregnant and have any of the following symptoms.

The Symptoms

- Loss of vision or blurred vision
- Queasiness
- Abdominal pains
- Sudden weight gain of more than 2lb in a week
- Dizziness
- Severe headaches

You should contact your doctor if you notice a sudden change. Keep in mind, however, that some of these symptoms are also associated with normal pregnancies.

Management of Pre-Eclampsia

If the baby is too immature for delivery doctors will try to manage the pre-eclampsia until a time when the baby can be safely delivered. If the baby is developed enough to allow delivery this is what the doctor may recommend, as the only way to treat pre-eclampsia is to deliver the baby.

Summing Up

- Different countries tend to have different definitions of normal blood pressure.

- In most countries a blood pressure greater than 140/90mmHg is considered to be elevated.

- If your blood pressure is greater than 160/100mmHg your doctor will advise treatment regardless of your cardiovascular risk.

- Your other risk factors for heart disease, angina and strokes will determine whether your blood pressure is treated if it's only mildly elevated.

- A high blood pressure during pregnancy can have serious consequences for mother and baby and requires the attention of a doctor.

- The hormone progesterone usually causes blood pressure to become decreased during pregnancy.

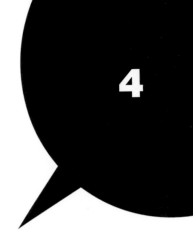

4

Why Do I Have High Blood Pressure?

Primary Hypertension

Wondering what the cause is when your doctor says there's something wrong with you is the logical thing to do. However, there is no known cause in the majority of instances of high blood pressure. It's just something that happens.

The blood pressure numbers don't increase all by themselves just because there's no known cause, though! There are many factors that could put you at risk of developing hypertension. Your blood vessels can go through many changes which have been associated with high blood pressure.

Which came first: The chicken or the egg? Just like the chicken and the egg, it can be difficult to work out if the changes in your blood vessels happened first, or if it was the high blood pressure that came first.

Risk Factors

- Family history of high blood pressure
- Drinking excessive amounts of alcohol
- Stressful lifestyle
- Excessive salt intake
- Being overweight

The only way to discover it is by having your blood pressure checked. There are no overt symptoms in most cases of hypertension, and no real underlying cause.

"Having one or more of these risk factors doesn't mean that you will definitely develop hypertension; they just make it more likely that at some point in your life you may develop it."

The Interaction between Hypertension, Cholesterol, Obesity and Diabetes

If your doctor diagnoses you with hypertension they will usually also look to see if you have diabetes or high cholesterol, as treating all of these conditions will reduce your risk of suffering from future heart disease or strokes. "Metabolic syndrome" is the name given to a condition which combines obesity, high blood pressure, high cholesterol and insulin resistance.

In recent times, the increase in prevalence of obesity has made this condition much more common. So what does metabolic syndrome mean?

If you have high blood pressure, insulin resistance, high cholesterol and a high body fat percentage, your risk of suffering from angina, stroke or heart attack is increased. If you have a combination of these problems, it's even higher.

The relation between the conditions that make up metabolic syndrome has not yet been figured out, so there's some controversy surrounding the idea of the syndrome. The name "Syndrome X" is preferred by some doctors, so no full agreement has been reached regarding the title. There is no doubt that this combination is bad for your health though, no matter what the doctors decide to call it.

Inessential Hypertension

This condition is also known as "Secondary Hypertension." Most of the time if there is an underlying cause this will be obvious to your doctor from asking you questions, taking a look at you and performing a few basic blood tests. Hypertension has an underlying cause in 5% of cases, and in these cases the high blood pressure is said to be *secondary* to the underlying issue.

Secondary hypertension can be caused by:

- Certain drugs and medicines
- CKD (chronic kidney disease)
- Coarctation of the aorta
- Hormone diseases

Unless your hypertension doesn't respond easily to treatment, your doctor is unlikely to look in great detail for an underlying cause, as the cause is usually obvious if there is one.

Symptoms of Secondary Hypertension

Unless you have symptoms related to the underlying cause, secondary hypertension usually has no symptoms. It is similar to primary hypertension in this regard.

Which Medications Can Cause Hypertension?

Medications do not often cause high blood pressure, though many can cause low blood pressure. Most of these medications will not cause you a problem if your blood pressure is normal to start with. Unfortunately, however, all medications have some side effects.

Hypertension can occur if you're taking...

- Certain painkillers
- Nasal decongestants
- Oral contraceptives
- Appetite Suppressants
- Recreational drugs
- Some herbal medications

"The combination of the following is termed the metabolic syndrome:

- Hypertension
- High cholesterol
- A tendency towards diabetes (called 'insulin resistance')
- A leaning towards being overweight, especially if the excess weight is around the abdomen."

- Migraine treatments
- Steroids

Many of these medications can be purchased at a chemist, which means that people often take them without consulting their doctor. You may require treatment for high blood pressure if taking these medications puts you into the "high" range. This can happen if your blood pressure is already in the upper range of normal.

Before you regularly take any of these medications, it's best to check with your doctor if your blood pressure is known to be "high" or "high normal".

Pain Killers

NSAIDS (Non-Steroidal Anti-Inflammatory Drugs) are the type of painkiller that can result in high blood pressure. Diclofenac, ibuprofen (also known as "Brufen") and aspirin all fall into this category.

Rather than using these NSAIDS, if you have high blood pressure try to use paracetamol if you need a painkiller.

Corticosteroids

"Cushing's Syndrome" is a condition that can occur as a result of long term steroid treatment. If you are on long-term steroid treatment your doctor will regularly monitor you for signs of Cushing's syndrome. Stretch marks, hypertension, a hump at the top of the back, excess hair growth and an increase in weight are all known symptoms of this condition.

You may take a regular steroid inhaler if you suffer from asthma. Steroids that are inhaled, however, are less likely to cause Cushing's syndrome than steroids taken in tablet form.

Decongestants

These are adrenaline like substances, for example "phenylephrine", which can increase your heart rate and narrow your arteries – both of which result in high blood pressure. Decongestants can often be found in medications used to treat colds and coughs. It shouldn't be a real problem for you to take these medications, however, unless you are already suffering from severe hypertension.

Treatments for Migraines

There are a variety of these medications. The blood vessels in your brain increase in diameter (dilate) during a migraine. Narrowing these blood vessels is how some medications work to treat the migraine.

Sumatriptan, Rizatriptan and other migraine treatments ending in "triptan" are generally the ones that work in this way. They have side effects like any other medication, though they are very effective in treating migraines. Increased blood pressure can be one of these side effects, as the medications narrow the blood vessels outside of the brain, as well of those in the brain.

Appetite Suppressants

All amphetamine based drugs can increase heart rate and blood pressure. The recreational drug "speed", or amphetamine, is the basis for many of the drugs that work to treat obesity by suppressing the appetite.

Oral Contraceptives

Increased blood pressure can be an issue for some people taking the combined oral contraceptive pill, which contains both oestrogen and progesterone. Your doctor will regularly check your blood pressure for this reason if you are on the pill.

High blood pressure often occurs as a result of the oestrogen pill. This means your doctor will probably suggest switching to the mini pill (also called the progesterone only pill) if your blood pressure rises when on the pill. Even when you are on the mini pill, however, your doctor will continue to keep an eye on your blood pressure as progesterone can also increase blood pressure in some women.

Herbal Medications

Herbal medicines that can increase blood pressure include:

- Panax ginseng
- Licorice
- St John's Wort

"Herbal medicines, just like prescribed medicines from your doctor, can have side effects and some herbal medicines, for example Ginseng and St Johns Wort, can increase blood pressure."

Many people who take herbal medications do so because they believe they won't cause any side effects, but side effects can occur as a result of any medication which has an effect on your body.

Hypertension can sometimes occur if you consume liquorice (licorice). If you are at risk of hypertension you should try not to consume too much liquorice. It's found in liquorice sticks and sweets, as well as some herbal medicines.

Illegal Substances

Dangerous effects on the heart and blood pressure are experienced by some people who use recreational drugs, such as methamphetamine (speed) and cocaine. These substances increase heart rate and blood pressure, which can be fatal in some instances.

Hormone Diseases and High Blood Pressure

The following hormone diseases can cause high blood pressure in some circumstances:

- Diabetes
- Primary aldosteronism
- Pheochromocytoma
- Hyperparathyroidism
- Over or under active thyroid
- Cushing's syndrome

Hypertension and Diabetes

High blood pressure can occur as a result of diabetes, which is often associated with changes in the blood vessels which make them stiff. Another cause of hypertension, kidney disease, can also occur as a result of diabetes.

Cushing's Syndrome

Taking steroid treatments can cause Cushing's syndrome, as discussed previously. Your adrenal glands can also produce steroids as natural hormones. Cushing's syndrome can occur if your adrenal glands produce too much steroid.

Primary Aldosteronism

Aldosterone is produced in the adrenal glands along with cortisol and is responsible for increasing the sodium level in your blood stream. If your body is producing too much of the hormone aldosterone, you are said to have Primary Aldosteronism (also known as Conn's syndrome and hyperaldosteronism). High blood pressure can occur as a result of this condition, as too much aldosterone leads to an increase of sodium in the bloodstream.

Over or Under Active Thyroid

High or low blood pressure can occur as a result of hypo (underactive) or hyper (overactive) thyroidism.

Pheochromocytoma

The hormones noradrenaline and adrenaline can be produced in too high a quantity if a growth called a pheochromocytoma develops in your adrenal glands. In normal amounts you won't notice any ill effects of these hormones, but if their levels are too high they have a similar effect to decongestant medication. They can also make you feel anxious or agitated.

Your heart rate and blood pressure can be increased by adrenaline and noradrenaline. When you feel stressed, these are the hormones responsible for increasing your heart rate.

Hyperparathyroidism

Overactive parathyroid glands are at the root of this condition. In medical terminology, "mara" means "next to" – these glands are next to the thyroid glands.

Calcium is similar to sodium in that it increases blood pressure. The levels of calcium in your bloodstream can be increased by overactive parathyroid glands.

Hypertension and Kidney Disease

Just as hypertension can lead to kidney disease, any kind of kidney disease can result in high blood pressure. If you have high blood pressure, then, your doctor will keep an eye on your kidney function, and if you have kidney disease your doctor will want to monitor your blood pressure.

Renovascular Hypertension

Atherosclerosis (fatty deposits building up in the walls of your arteries) are usually the cause of this condition, in which the blood vessels ("vascular") supplying one or both of your kidneys ("reno") become narrower. Your kidneys are unable to get enough blood as a result. So that more blood flows to the kidneys, they will attempt to increase your blood pressure.

Hypertension and Obesity

29% of adults in the UK are obese – an increase from 26% in 2016. Obesity is not healthy – though the statistics do suggest that it's becoming the norm.

Why Do Overweight People Have Higher Blood Pressure?

As your weight increases your heart and blood vessels have to work harder to supply your cells with the oxygen and nutrients that they need. As a general rule, the heart of someone of "healthy" weight won't have to work as hard as the heart of someone of the same height who is overweight, when it comes to transporting blood around the body. Your blood pressure, then, will increase as you gain weight.

Sleep Apnea

Symptoms of sleep apnea include:

- Snoring loudly
- Feeling tired when you're awake
- Times when you stop breathing in the night

In sleep apnea the air passages to the lungs become blocked when you fall asleep. Sleep apnea can also occur as a result of obesity. It causes the individual to stop breathing entirely several times throughout the night ("apnea" means that breathing has stopped), and to snore loudly when they are breathing. In the long term, it can lead to an increase in blood pressure and damage to blood vessels as it results in a lack of oxygen in the bloodstream.

> "Obesity is a major public health problem, both internationally and within the UK. Being overweight or obese is associated with an increased risk of a number of common diseases and causes of premature death, including diabetes, cardiovascular disease and some cancers."
>
> The Nuffield Trust

Coarctation of the Aorta and High Blood Pressure

Blood pressure, especially in the arms, can be increased when the main blood vessel (aorta) which carries blood from your heart to the rest of your body is narrowed – a condition called "Coarctation of the Aorta". Although it often isn't detected until much later in life, this is a condition that people are born with.

Treating Inessential Hypertension

Treating the underlying cause will usually cure secondary hypertension.

Summing Up

- Primary hypertension, where there are risk factors but no underlying causes, is the most common form of high blood pressure.
- Rarely, hypertension has an underlying cause and is termed "secondary hypertension".
- Once the underlying cause is treated, the high blood pressure usually returns to normal.

How Hypertension Affects You

How hypertension is going to affect your health will probably be one of your first concerns following diagnosis. The ways in which your health will be affected by hypertension will be discussed in this chapter.

Symptoms

High blood pressure can be a particularly frustrating condition. In many cases, symptoms will only become apparent after the damage has been done, and without getting tested it can remain unnoticed until that point.

No Symptoms at All

The majority of people with hypertension will feel perfectly normal, having no idea that they have the condition. General check-ups and doctors visits for other ailments are usually where high blood pressure is first noticed for this reason. Because there are no symptoms of high blood pressure the damage that it causes is often not recognised until it is too late.

I Have Nosebleeds – Do I Have Hypertension?

Not necessarily! Nosebleeds are not more common amongst people with high blood pressure. Most people with nosebleeds have a perfectly normal blood, though many people believe that nosebleeds are caused by high blood pressure. It seems like a logical explanation, but it simply isn't the case.

How about Headaches?

A muzzy, confused feeling in the head, blurred vision and, yes, a headache can all occur if you have very high blood pressure (also known as "malignant hypertension"). That said, this is very uncommon and the majority of headaches have nothing to do with hypertension.

If It Causes No Symptoms, Why Does Blood Pressure Matter?

This question is fairly common. High blood pressure can cause damage to organs in the body such as the kidneys, brain, eyes and heart, so even though people with high blood pressure feel well they are dealing with a big problem.

The Effects of Hypertension on the Blood Vessels

Blood flows through your blood vessels in a similar way to water flowing through pipes. However, unlike pipes, blood vessels are flexible. Your blood vessels carry out the vital task of carrying blood from your heart to cells all over your body. In response to the needs of your body, they can change their shape to adjust the amount of blood flowing through them.

"Often described as a 'silent killer' because it rarely causes symptoms, high blood pressure was responsible for around 75,000 deaths in 2015, according to the Global Burden of Disease report."

GOV.UK

Arterial Stiffness

Unlike pipes, blood vessels don't usually burst under pressure, but they do stiffen and lose their flexibility under the continual onslaught of blood rushing through them at high pressure. If the pressure of the blood flowing through them is too high, blood vessels can become damaged – just like the pipes in a central heating system can get damaged if the water pressure is too high.

Atherosclerosis – Fatty Blood Vessels

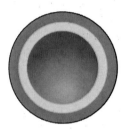 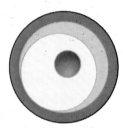 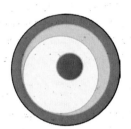

| Normal artery | Fat starts to build up in artery wall | Artery blocked by blood clot |

"High blood pressure doesn't just make blood vessels stiff, it can also damage their lining and trigger a process called atherosclerosis – which is similar to a scar forming inside the blood vessel."

The Greek word for a lump of wax gives us the term "atheroma". "Sclerosis", meanwhile, comes from the word for "scar".

The centre of the artery becomes narrow when fat builds up on the scars of their damaged lining. This means that less oxygen – and the blood that carries it – can get to where it is needed in the body, as it becomes difficult for blood to flow through the affected blood vessel. The blood vessel can even become blocked by a blood clot in very severe cases, meaning that no blood or oxygen can pass through it at all.

Symptoms of Atherosclerosis

The following symptoms are commonly caused by atherosclerosis:

- Chest pain
- Reduced blood supply to brain (stroke)
- CKD (chronic kidney disease)
- Leg ulcers

- Heart attacks

Angina occurs when the heart doesn't have enough oxygen but there is still some blood getting through the artery. Angina, or chest pain, is one of the best known symptoms of a lack of oxygen, though the symptoms of atherosclerosis will vary depending on which part of your body is being starved of oxygen. If the blood vessel supplying the brain or heart becomes completely blocked off, a stroke or heart attack will occur.

The next section will discuss heart attacks, strokes and angina in greater detail.

Hypertension and the Heart

There are two main ways that hypertension can affect your heart. It can lead to the enlargement of the heart muscle, and can cause heart attacks and angina if blockages occur in the blood vessels supplying the heart muscle.

Cardiomegaly

High blood pressure means that the pressure in your blood vessels is greater than normal, and your heart has to work harder to pump against this pressure. The heart's job is to pump blood through the blood vessels – it's essentially just a pump made of muscle.

Your heart becomes larger and more muscular as a result of this extra work. It's sort of like someone having really big leg or arm muscles as a result of working out in the gym.

Surely an Increase in Muscle Is a Good Thing?

Serious health problems can unfortunately occur as a result of an increase in muscle in your heart (called "cardiomegaly" or "hypertrophy" by doctors). The following are the three main issues with an increase in heart muscle:

- The heart can't pump as effectively as before, as it becomes stiff as it enlarges.

- Angina can occur as a bigger blood supply is needed by the extra muscle, and the blood vessels supplying the heart can't always deliver it.

- The extra muscle puts a strain on the nerves that trigger the regular pumping of the heart, if these nerves malfunction the heart can beat irregularly which can be life threatening.

Chest Pain (Angina Pectoris)

'Pectoris' comes from the Latin for chest. The Greek word for "strangling" gives us the word "angina".

Angina can occur if the blood supply to the heart is unable to keep up with oxygen demands, but it most commonly occurs when atherosclerosis causes the blood vessels supplying the heart to become narrowed. It can happen if the heart is more muscular than it should be, or if it is beating very quickly.

Common Symptoms of Angina

- Chest feels tight or heavy
- Struggling to catch your breath
- Nausea

These symptoms may also be signalling that you're suffering from a heart attack. If you suffer from angina and normal treatment is not relieving the symptoms, talk to your doctor immediately.

The Heart Attack

Oxygen supply to the heart can return to normal even after it is reduced during angina. In heart attacks, however, part of the heart actually dies because the blood vessels are totally blocked and the oxygen is completely prevented from reaching an area of the heart muscle.

Symptoms of a Heart Attack

- Chest feels tight or heavy
- Struggling to catch your breath
- Loss of consciousness
- Sweating
- Nausea and vomiting

If you or somebody you know has these symptoms call a doctor immediately so proper treatment can be given quickly. Severe angina attacks and heart attacks can have very similar symptoms.

"Angina pectoris (abbreviated to 'angina') is the name given to the pain in the chest caused by a lack of oxygen getting to the heart muscle."

The Brain and High Blood Pressure

If your brain is starved of oxygen for even a short time your brain tissue will die quickly. Your risk of suffering a stroke can be increased if you have high blood pressure, as the blood vessels supplying the brain can become blocked.

If there is a lack of oxygen to the part of your brain that controls movement of your right arm then this arm becomes paralysed. Similarly, it will become difficult to speak if the part of your brain that controls speech is starved of oxygen. The blood vessel that is blocked will determine which stroke symptoms you exhibit, as there are a number of blood vessels that supply different areas of the brain.

- A stroke that lasts less than 24 hours is known as a TIA
- Patients can recover well from a stroke with time and physiotherapy
- Repeated small strokes over a number of years can cause dementia
- Many strokes last for more than 24 hours

Symptoms of Stroke

If you or anyone you know has these symptoms you need to call a doctor as soon as possible so that the stroke can be treated.

- Face or limbs suddenly becoming weak
- Mixing words
- Sudden inability to find correct words

The Eyes and High Blood Pressure

Your eyes can be affected by high blood pressure, though many people don't realise it.

Hypertension doesn't often cause problems with vision. There are a lot of small blood vessels in the back of your eye. It's actually pretty easy to see these blood vessels – and the eye is the only part of the body where this is the case. This means your doctor might want to check your eyes if you have hypertension, just to see how your blood vessels are being affected.

Hypertension and the Kidneys

Blood is continuously forced through small blood vessels in the kidneys and waste products are 'squeezed' out of them and into a collection of tubes that join up to drain into your bladder. Many of the waste substances produced in your body are removed by your kidneys.

Squeezing waste products through the blood vessels can become difficult in patients with hypertension, as the walls of their blood vessels become thicker. Eventually, the waste products will build up in the patient's body as their kidneys can no longer remove them efficiently.

Kidney Failure

Also known as 'renal failure', kidney failure is the term used when your kidneys are no longer able to function properly. Usually, high blood pressure is detected and treated a long time before renal failure happens.

Removing waste products in severe cases of kidney failure can require dialysis, otherwise the waste products can build up to dangerous levels. Your bloodstream can then have its waste products filtered out, as dialysis essentially carries out the job of the kidney.

Your doctor will want to take a regular blood test to keep an eye on your kidney function, but if your blood pressure is well treated your kidneys will not usually become damaged.

Are There Other Ways in which Hypertension Affects the Kidneys?

This has also been discussed in Chapter 4 under the heading 'renovascular hypertension'.

The kidneys are supplied by large blood vessels, and hypertension can do some damage if it blocks these vessels. When this happens, the kidneys work to increase the amount of blood they receive by releasing hormones, having sensed that there isn't enough blood flowing through them to properly remove the body's waste. These hormones increase the blood pressure even more, which can cause further problems.

Can Other Parts of My Body Be Damaged by High Blood Pressure?

Atherosclerosis is the main way in which damage is caused by high blood pressure. For example, if the arteries to your legs start to become blocked leg ulcers can result. Blockages can occur in any artery affected by atherosclerosis, but the main organs affected are the heart and the brain.

My Doctor Talks about Cardiovascular Disease, What Is This?

The aim of treating or preventing hypertension is to reduce your risk of cardiovascular disease (or 'cardiovascular risk'). Although hypertension can cause atherosclerosis in all arteries, the main ones that doctors are concerned about are those supplying the heart and brain. Sometimes they include blockages of the arteries supplying the legs and kidneys under the heading 'cardiovascular disease'.

Doctors are usually referring to disease of the blood vessels and heart due to fatty deposits in the arteries (atherosclerosis) when they talk about cardiovascular disease. In most cases, they're talking about heart attacks, stroke and angina when they discuss this in relation to high blood pressure.

Doctors are usually referring to the following conditions when discussing cardiovascular disease:

- Heart attack
- Stroke
- Angina

Cardiovascular Risk Factors

Other risk factors include:

- Unhealthy diet
- Smoking tobacco
- Diabetes

The problems mentioned in this chapter have a number of risk factors, and hypertension is just one of them.

If you have multiple risk factors for cardiovascular disease, they are multiplied together, rather than simply added. This means that your risk of developing cardiovascular disease is higher than the sum of the individual risks if you have all of these factors.

Smoking

Around one in five people in the UK smoke. However, as of 2018, 60% of smokers say they intend to quit and more than 1 in 8 are planning to quit in the next 3 months.

It's important that you try to give up smoking if you want to avoid suffering from any of these conditions in the future – though it won't be easy.

"Smoking is the biggest contributor to suffering cardiovascular disease and it greatly magnifies the risk from high blood pressure."

Summing Up

- Hypertension is a disease that affects all parts of your body – it's not just a matter of a couple of abnormal numbers.

- Hypertension can cause renal failure and damage to the kidneys, as well as angina, strokes and heart attacks.

- Taking treatment to reduce your blood pressure will reduce the risk of these diseases.

- Your doctor will advise that you also treat your diabetes and/or high cholesterol, as these amplify the risks associated with high blood pressure.

- Smoking is the biggest culprit of all when it comes to causing heart disease and strokes, therefore, if you are told you have high blood pressure, diabetes or high cholesterol it is very important that you try to stop smoking.

- The problem is that because you can't feel that you have high blood pressure it can cause damage without you even noticing.

6

Low Blood Pressure: Causes and Treatment

This chapter will discuss what low blood pressure is and whether it is a real problem. Usually, people are referring to their blood pressure being too high when they mention problems with blood pressure. Many people will be told that their blood pressure is low, but this is usually nothing to worry about, in fact many doctors would say it is something to aim for.

Low blood pressure often occurs in people who are fit and active and they suffer no ill effects of this. But low blood pressure can also be an issue.

How Low Is Too Low?

"Hypotension" is the term used when someone's blood pressure is too low. "Tension" refers to pressure, while "hypo" means "low".

Your risk of suffering from strokes or heart attacks will generally get lower the lower your blood pressure is.

Some people with low blood pressure can end up dealing with symptoms, however, and dangerously low blood pressure may occur on rare occasions. One of the most common symptoms of a low blood pressure is fainting.

Hypotension Symptoms

"A low blood pressure is defined as a systolic reading of less than 90mmHg or a diastolic less than 60mmHg."

Blood flow to your organs through your arteries will be reduced if your blood pressure becomes too low. Although the majority of your body's organs will be able to deal with a brief reduction in blood supply, the brain needs more energy than the other organs in your body and will not be able to cope with reduced blood supply. So, your brain is very sensitive to a reduction in blood pressure.

It needs more blood to deliver nutrients and oxygen than other vital organs do.

Your brain failing to get enough blood is the cause of the majority of symptoms of low blood pressure. A person may slump to the floor in a faint if they're suffering from hypotension. If they are left lying down, people who have fainted usually recover quickly, although they may feel a little sick and drowsy for a while afterwards. Blood flow usually recovers rapidly once they are lying down, as blood doesn't have to fight against gravity to get to the brain.

These are the main symptoms of hypotension:

- Lightheadedness
- Vision issues
- Feeling cold
- Fatigue
- Difficulty concentrating
- Nausea
- Fainting

These symptoms may also occur with other conditions (for example, the common cold), so having these symptoms doesn't necessarily mean you have hypotension. Low blood pressure is not the only explanation for having these symptoms.

Is It a Fit or a Faint?

Onlookers will sometimes confuse a faint with a fit, as people who have fainted can have some jerky movements in their limbs. A faint is not usually accompanied by the other cardinal symptoms of a fit, though, and the jerky movements won't generally last as long as they would with a fit.

A fit's cardinal symptoms include:

- Urination
- Fatigue, even after the person has recovered
- Loss of control of the bowels

People who have fainted have been brought around using "smelling salts" - which release ammonia gas - since Roman times. These are believed to increase alertness by irritating the lining of the nose in order to stimulate breathing.

Hypotension Causes

Your doctor will usually only start looking for a cause to your low blood pressure if it's causing you problems - in most cases, hypotension has no underlying cause and isn't a major issue. Your doctor will usually take things further if your dizziness or fainting become frequent or start affecting your ability to go about your normal life, but feeling dizzy or fainting every now and then will not generally warrant further investigation.

An underlying condition may be causing your hypotension. Potential causes may include...

- Being dehydrated
- Low iron levels or bleeding
- Being pregnant
- Cardiovascular disease and other heart conditions
- Orthostatic hypotension

"Fainting is a sudden, temporary loss of consciousness that usually results in a fall. Healthcare professionals often use the term 'syncope' when referring to fainting because it distinguishes fainting from other causes of temporary unconsciousness, such as seizures (fits) or concussion."

Health Service Executive (HSE)

- Post prandial hypotension
- Medications
- Endocrine (Hormone) abnormalities
- Severe allergy (anaphylaxis)
- Infections

Dehydration

Frequent causes of dehydration are:

- Not drinking enough
- Gastroenteritis and diarrhoea
- Sweating too much (e.g. during a workout)
- Diuretic medications
- Sunburn
- Vomiting

Hypotension is often caused by dehydration.

What many people don't realise is that losing water isn't the only issue when you become dehydrated. Athletes often drink specially made solutions of water and salts when they are training or competing. Sweat contains water and salts, and you need to replace both of these - not just the water. Most people out and about in the heat don't need to buy special solutions but just need to drink juices as well as plain water.

If water is replaced independently of salt, the salts that remain in your body become dilute. If you become dehydrated as a result of vomiting or diarrhoea, you will also be losing water and salts. Many people die as a result of drinking too much water without also replacing salts, which can lead to serious illness. If you need to replace salt and water after vomiting or diarrhoea, you can by special salt and water solutions from pharmacies and fitness shops which will do the job.

Anyone may become dehydrated, but the condition is especially dangerous for young children and older adults.

"On a hot day it is easy to lose water through sweat without even knowing it. Dehydration is even more pronounced if you are exercising in the heat. It is therefore important to increase your fluid intake on a hot day to avoid becoming dehydrated."

Anaphylaxis, Infections and Bleeding

Hospital treatment will be necessary if your hypotension is a result of more serious conditions. That you are not well will be quickly noticed by both you and your doctor, as these conditions are generally pretty obvious. Bleeding is the exception to this, however. Blood can be lost slowly during menstruation or through the gut so while blood loss will sometimes be obvious, this is not always the case.

Your blood count can fall significantly before you experience any symptoms if you lose the blood gradually. Before offering treatment, if your symptoms are due to gradual blood loss, your doctor will need to investigate the case. An urgent blood transfusion may, however, be advised if you have lost a lot of blood.

Pregnancy

To ensure that enough blood is reaching the growing embryo, changes occur in the circulatory system during pregnancy. The hormone progesterone causes blood pressure to fall, with the most significant change in pressure occurring in the second trimester of pregnancy (12 to 27 weeks).

The blood pressure can also drop suddenly sometimes when a heavily pregnant person lies down. To prevent this from occurring, after about 20 weeks into pregnancy, women should not lie down flat and will normally sleep with a pillow under their side. Large veins are responsible for taking blood back to the heart, and blood pressure can be affected when the weight of the growing foetus puts pressure on these veins.

If a pregnant person faints, they should be allowed to lie down with a pillow under one side until they have recovered.

Low Blood Count

If your doctor finds that you are anaemic they will find out the cause behind this before offering you treatment. Blood loss is often the cause for anaemia, or low blood count. Bone marrow that fails to produce enough blood cells can also be a cause. Dietary deficiencies of vitamins like folate or B12, or minerals like iron, are a common cause, though there are many other reasons a low blood count may occur.

Pale skin is one of the main indicators of anaemia. Though many other factors may cause this pallor. The main issue with anaemia is that it means not enough oxygen is able to reach your body's tissues and organs.

"Red blood cells are given their colour by a red pigment called haemoglobin – this pigment is also responsible for transporting oxygen around the body. So when there is a lack of red blood cells, there is also a shortage of haemoglobin – and not enough oxygen is delivered to the various tissues and organs."

Irish Health

Hormone Disorders Causing Low Blood Pressure

Most of the time people with a hormone disorder will know that they have this before a low blood pressure is found. Hypotension can be caused by the following common hormone disorders:

- Diabetes
- Addison's disease
- Hyper-/Hypothyroidism

Hormone disorders are not often diagnosed in people suffering from hypotension. Addison's disease, a condition where the hormones that normally keep your blood pressure up are not produced in high enough quantities by the adrenal glands, is an exception to this rule. Your doctor may want to test you for Addison's disease if your low blood pressure is causing issues.

Cardiovascular Disease and Other Heart Conditions

Low blood pressure can occur as a result of both heart disease and the medications used to treat heart disease. Hypotension can also often be caused by cardiac (or heart) failure. The medications commonly used to treat heart failure can also cause low blood pressure. Heart failure often occurs after suffering from heart attacks. In this condition, the muscle of the heart becomes weaker and is not able to generate the force it needs to pump the blood properly.

Suffering from hypotension for many years or having an irregular heartbeat can also result in heart failure.

Your doctor will have to balance keeping your blood pressure up with treating your heart failure if you have the two conditions.

Common Medications That Can Cause a Low Blood Pressure

- Medications that cause dehydration and water loss (diuretics)
- Certain medications for depression
- Sildenafil (viagra)
- Some treatments for schizophrenia
- Any treatment for high blood pressure

Orthostatic Hypotension

A drop in blood pressure when you stand up is very common. This is because the force of gravity means that blood pools in the veins in your legs and less blood flows back to your heart and from there to your brain. Low blood pressure related to posture is known as orthostatic, or postural, hypotension. Postural hypotension is more common in people who are prone to low blood pressure and people over 65 years old.

Post Prandial Hypotension

Post prandial hypotension is more common in people who have high blood pressure and people who are on medications for blood pressure.

In order to carry out the task of digesting and absorbing your food, your intestines and stomach need a high volume of blood when you eat. Some of your blood vessels will restrict to compensate for this, and your heart rate will increase – the same mechanisms that kick into action when you stand up. Your blood pressure may drop after eating if this doesn't happen to a large enough extent.

'Post' means after and 'prandial' means eating. So, post prandial hypotension means low blood pressure after eating.

Activity: Work with your family to learn how the body tries to avoid postural and post prandial hypotension.

1 Lie down for 5 minutes and get someone to take your pulse.

2 Stand up quickly, wait for a minute and check your pulse again. Standing up should result in an increased heart rate.

3 Checking your pulse before and after eating should yield similar results.

Do I Need to Go to the Doctor for Hypotension?

If your symptoms are just occasional, for example when you are dehydrated or if you have got up too quickly, then your doctor will probably not take things any further. If you're experiencing troublesome symptoms as a result of or alongside your low blood pressure, it's worth looking into it in greater detail. If there is no obvious underlying reason your doctor will examine you and investigate to make sure there is no serious underlying cause.

Investigations for Low Blood Pressure

If you are on medications that lower blood pressure, are pregnant or have heart disease then you already know why you have hypotension.

If you have hypotension and don't know why, your doctor may carry out investigations such as...

- ECG (heart tracing)
- Checking for hormone disorders or anaemia through blood tests
- Checking for abnormal heart rhythms through 24-hour Holter monitoring
- An ultrasound of your heart – to see if it is pumping properly
- A 24 hour blood pressure monitor

Treating Hypotension

There are medications that can be used to increase your blood pressure, but as with all medications these have side effects and you and your doctor will need to work out whether the side effects from the medications are better than suffering symptoms from low blood pressure.

Treatment of the underlying cause is usually a key part of treating hypotension. The blood pressure will go back to normal, for example, if thyroid disease is causing the problem and the thyroid disease is successfully treated. If your blood pressure is low because of medications you are taking, your doctor will try to adjust these to return to healthy blood pressure.

In some cases, the cause will have no suitable treatment or the doctor will be unable to find an underlying cause.

Summing Up

- Unless it is causing too many symptoms, low blood pressure is generally seen as a good thing.

- Most people with low blood pressure will experience only temporary symptoms which are often associated with dehydration.

- Finding and treating the cause is generally the best treatment for low blood pressure.

- If your symptoms from low blood pressure are troublesome your doctor will look for the cause of this.

- The most common symptoms from having low blood pressure are faints and dizziness.

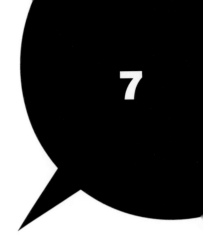

7

Lifestyle Changes to Treat Hypertension

A number of questions may come to mind when you hear you have high blood pressure…

- How will my life change?
- How long will treatment last?
- What can I do to help?
- Can I lead a normal life with hypertension?
- Will I have to take medications?

Lifestyle measures that can reduce your blood pressure – changes you can make and things that can stay the same – will be covered in this chapter. In the next chapter, we'll cover the more medical treatments which should be used alongside these lifestyle changes.

Will High Blood Pressure Stop Me Living an Active Life?

"If you live a fit and active life, being told you have high blood pressure shouldn't stop you doing any of your usual activities. However, if you enjoy some sports, like scuba diving, you may need to tell any clubs that you are involved in about your condition."

No way! Becoming more active is actually one of the things many doctors will encourage people with hypertension to do.

"Malignant hypertension", or very high blood pressure, is the one exception to this rule. Your doctor will recommend that you start taking medications to lower your blood pressure if you have malignant hypertension, and you'll be asked to go into hospital for a period of rest. Most people with hypertension won't have to go to hospital, however, as malignant hypertension is very rare.

Getting your family involved in your treatment and keeping them in the loop is generally a good idea if you're diagnosed with high blood pressure. You'll feel less isolated, and they'll feel less worried about your health.

If your blood pressure isn't well controlled, it's advised that you shouldn't go scuba diving or participate in similar activities.

Exercise to Reduce Blood Pressure

If you have mild hypertension you may find that increasing the amount of exercise you do will lower your blood pressure without the need for treatment. A sedentary lifestyle is one of the key risk factors for hypertension. Exercise will reduce your risk of heart attacks and strokes and keep you in good shape, even if it doesn't dramatically reduce your blood pressure.

Which Exercise Is Best for Me?

It can be a bit of a shock to the system for those who have got out of the habit of exercising, however, it is surprising how quickly you can incorporate exercise into your daily routine and even start to enjoy it.

- Think about the forms of exercise you might enjoy, and sign up for one of those
- Stick with it, even if it's difficult
- Start off gradually

According to the guidelines, healthy adults under the age of 65 should aim for one of two exercise plans…

- Vigorous exercise for 20 minutes a day on three days of the week

Or

- 5 days a week, participate in at least 30 minutes of exercise that makes you break into a sweat or raises your heart rate without making it difficult to talk.

Remember to start gradually, but not so gradually that you'll end up grinding to a halt at the smallest opportunity. If you do give up, even for one day, it is easy to sit back in your armchair and forget about your exercise program. If you are fit and healthy there is no reason why you can't build up to full strength after a week or two. Starting either of these programs will be tough if you haven't done any exercise in a long time.

As Plato once said, "Lack of activity destroys the good condition of every human being, while movement and methodical physical exercise save it and preserve it."

If you hate going out in the rain jogging is probably not the exercise for you, however, if you like social events, why not join a badminton group? Giving up is not an option here. If you're likely to find excuses not to do a certain form of exercise, pick one that's not so easy to avoid.

There's a good chance that your children may also develop hypertension if you or your parents have it. Try and get your kids involved in your exercise problem to minimise their likelihood of developing future problems. Children are more likely to stay fit and healthy and enjoy exercise later on if they grow up thinking it's a normal part of life.

"The important thing about exercise is that it is enjoyable. It is no use dragging yourself off to the swimming pool three times a week if you hate getting wet."

Think about Getting a Dog

A dog is a fantastic family pet and they really do have to be walked, so if you have high blood pressure a dog will mean that you can't make any excuses not to exercise. If dedicating time to walkies is the only thing stopping you from getting a dog, you should definitely consider adopting one.

Your blood pressure may also be helped by the opportunity walking a dog will give you to look around and relax outdoors.

How Will Other Medical Conditions Affect This?

You shouldn't generally run into any difficulties if you start building up your exercise program gradually. Ask your doctor for guidance if you're worried about doing too much too quickly or have had a heart attack or angina in the past.

Smoking and Blood Pressure

"Although you can generally carry on with life as normal if you have high blood pressure, if you smoke you should really consider stopping. The US Surgeon General has called smoking 'the leading preventable cause of disease and deaths in the United States'."

Many people associate smoking with lung cancer, but it is also one of the major causes of cardiovascular disease.

Smoking is a major issue in the United Kingdom. If you have hypertension, smoking will cut an average of 10 years off your life expectancy. Your risk of suffering from a heart attack, stroke or angina is significantly increased if you combine smoking with high blood pressure.

What's more, hypertension is a condition that's at least partly hereditary, so if you have high blood pressure there's a strong likelihood your children will also develop it later on. Similarly, children are more likely to grow up to be smokers if they saw their parents smoking. This means your children are more likely to suffer from cardiovascular disease when they grow up if you smoke and have high blood pressure.

You can help to prevent your children from taking up this habit when they grow up if you stop smoking today. This is really important because, other than getting them to exercise regularly, there's very little you can do to reduce their risk of developing hypertension.

Giving Up Smoking

- Identify your reason for quitting
- Ask your friends and family for support
- Look into nicotine patches and similar devices
- Ask your GP for advice
- Keep away from situations in which you would normally smoke
- Pick a date

It is sometimes better to get together with a group of friends who also want to quit – then you can support each other. Giving up smoking can be a real struggle, so you need to identify your reason for quitting and use that as your source of motivation. Many people's reason is their health in the future, but yours can be something else. You might also be thinking of the future health of your children, your ability to play football at the weekend or just the smell of it in your house.

Choose the date you're going to stop smoking, and stick to it. Don't allow yourself to push it back a week or a month, no matter how much you fancy a cigarette.

Often smoking is just as much a habit as an addiction and to break the habit you have to break from your normal smoking pattern. Taking yourself away from the situations where you would normally smoke is the most important thing you can do in the first few months. If you usually smoke when you go to the bar with friends, consider not going to the bar. Try socialising in the daytime instead, at a café, for example.

Many people who are addicted to nicotine find nicotine replacement therapies like patches and gum to be very helpful. If you need any additional advice, go and talk to your GP – they'll be delighted you're quitting and will have lots of advice and resources to offer you.

What to Eat to Lower Your Blood Pressure

One major contributor to hypertension is sodium chloride, or salt. One of the main reasons that Westerners' blood pressure increases as they age is that our diets contain huge amounts of salt. We certainly don't need to add salt to our food. We don't need to eat any more salt than is found naturally in a balanced, healthy diet, but many of us add it to our food out of habit or because they like the taste.

When scientists studied tribal societies in areas like Papua New Guinea, they discovered that the elders of these societies had blood pressure that was no higher than that of the younger members. Until then, it was believed that increased blood pressure with age was normal and unavoidable. The people in these tribes didn't add salt to their food, and it is believed that this is the reason for their healthier blood pressure.

How Much Salt Should I Be Eating?

You don't have to add any salt to your food to get enough salt in your diet.

- Each day, we shouldn't consume any more than 2.4 grams (one teaspoon) of salt
- The food on your table doesn't need any added salt
- You should not need to add any salt to your cooking

Sodium chloride, or salt, is found in all foods – meat, vegetables and even fruit.

'To cease smoking is the easiest thing I ever did. I ought to know because I've done it a thousand times.'

Attributed to Mark Twain

Going Salt Free

"Most people will have got used to a large amount of salt in their diet and will find that cutting this out completely can make their meals taste bland. Rather than go cold turkey gradually reduce the amount of salt you add to your food, both when you cook and at the table."

Gradually reduce the amount of salt in your whole family's diet, this will be healthier for all of you and it will mean that the person who cooks doesn't have to make separate meals. Your meals will taste perfectly lovely if you gradually reduce the amount of salt to nothing over a few weeks. Because hypertension is often associated with high cholesterol and diabetes you should also try to cut down on fatty or sugary foods.

What to Cut Out

These foods should gradually be removed from your diet…

- Table and cooking salt
- Non-organic foods
- Foods that are high in sugar
- Fatty foods
- Ready prepared meals

To help them taste nicer while keeping production costs low, processed foods, meals eaten out and microwave meals tend to have a high salt content. If you look at the packets, many will tell you how much salt the product contains. A lot of food manufacturers are trying to cut down on the amount of salt in their products, so cutting down shouldn't be too tricky!

That said, it's best to try and avoid processed food and microwave meals altogether as they can make it difficult to work out your total amount of salt for the day.

Foods to Eat

Information about the DASH diet can be found at: **www.dashdiet.org**.

You should aim for a healthy diet with at least five portions of fruit or veg per day if you have hypertension (or if your blood pressure is normal). You may be able to avoid having to take medication for blood pressure if you follow the DASH (Dietary Approaches to Stop Hypertension) dietary eating plan if your blood pressure is only slightly high.

If you do have to take medications, following the DASH eating plan may still lower your blood pressure somewhat and reduce the amount of medication you need.

Cooking is a great way of spending time with your family; it will also help to get your kids interested in eating a healthy diet when they get older. Try to spend at least three nights per week eating and cooking healthy meals together if you have a family.

Hypertension and Alcohol

If you are a heavy drinker with high blood pressure reducing the amount you drink to a moderate amount can be almost as effective as taking one of the medications that your doctor may recommend you take for your blood pressure. Many people aren't aware that alcohol can increase your blood pressure – though most will have heard that a glass of red wine is good for the health.

You're unlikely to have any real difficulties if you follow the NHS guidelines for alcohol units, which advise that you…

- should drink no more than 14 units of alcohol per week (men and women)

- try to have a few drink-free days every week

- spread your drinking over 3 or more days if you regularly drink as much as 14 units a week

The recommended 14 units is the equivalent to 10 small glasses of low-strength wine or six pints of average-strength beer.

Your blood pressure may be increased dramatically if you consume higher levels of alcohol than this.

Stress and Blood Pressure

What Does Stress Mean?

Non medical people often use the word stress to describe a situation that they have little control over or which worries them in some way. The hormones that your body would normally use to help you get out of a tricky situation is produced in greater amounts when you are under stress. Noradrenalin, cortisol and adrenalin and the hormones produced in this reaction.

"Once you get into the swing of eating healthily it gets easier to prepare tasty meals, but if you need inspiration, there is a diet called the DASH (Dietary Approaches to Stop Hypertension) diet which has been proven in properly conducted scientific studies to reduce blood pressure."

In the short term the release of these hormones causes your blood pressure to increase. They get your body to pump more blood that's rich in oxygen and glucose to your muscles, getting them ready to run. Whether you're being shouted at by your boss or being chased by a pack of wild dogs, the chemical reaction that happens in your body is the same.

What Does Stress Have to Do with Blood Pressure?

In most cases, your blood pressure will fall back to normal levels when the hormones are reduced after the stressful situation is resolved. But some stressful situations can last a while, and that can be a problem.

'Stress is an ignorant state. It believes that everything is an emergency.'

Natalie Goldberg, author of Wild Mind

If Short Term Stress Puts Up Blood Pressure, Can Long Term Stress Do the Same?

Doctors know that long term stress is associated with hypertension, but whether stress directly causes hypertension is not known. It's difficult to work out for certain whether long-term stress can lead to increased blood pressure that lasts longer than the high blood pressure caused by short-term stress, however logical it seems.

Other risk factors of hypertension – such as drinking too much, not getting enough exercise, gaining weight and eating poorly – are often present in those who are stressed. Doctors are yet to figure out if high blood pressure is caused by the stress or the risk factors that tend to be linked with it.

Should I Avoid Stressful Situations if I Have High Blood Pressure?

There's no real point in telling people to avoid stress, as most people have no real control over whether or not they are put in stressful situations. You can, however, make your stress a little easier to deal with if you do things that make you feel better about yourself and your life. If you want to cope with stress, the most tried and tested way of doing this is by engaging in regular exercise, as this can lower your cortisol levels.

Coping with difficult situations can also be easier if you have better self esteem, which you can work towards by drinking less, investing more time in your interests and eating healthily.

Summing Up

- Many people believe that being diagnosed with high blood pressure means you'll have to take tablets for the rest of your life, so finding out you have this condition can be a little upsetting.

- However, there are many things that you can do along with your family to try to reduce your blood pressure without going anywhere near a pharmacy.

- These measures should also reduce your stress levels at the same time as combating your high blood pressure.

- Stress and high blood pressure go together.

- However, there is some evidence that relaxation techniques may reduce blood pressure.

- You may not need any additional treatment if you're eating healthily, reaching a healthier weight, drinking less and exercising regularly, as all of these things can reduce blood pressure.

8

Treatments for Hypertension

After reading this chapter you should have enough information about the treatments and potential side effects to allow you to enter into a discussion with your doctor about what is best for you.

Many people with high blood pressure will not have suffered any ill effects from it, and will display no symptoms. They'll generally feel perfectly well. This means that you may be a little reluctant to take medications when you're initially diagnosed with high blood pressure, and it's likely that you'll want some information about the drugs you're being encouraged to take.

Medicines that Treat High Blood Pressure

- Reducing your blood pressure to <140/<85 is the goal of hypertension treatments
- Different people work better with different medications
- There are many different types of medication to treat hypertension
- These medications are grouped into categories depending on how they work

What Different Types of Medication Are There?

"Antihypertensives", or antihypertensive medications, is the name given to medications that treat hypertension.

The following are the main categories of medication used to treat hypertension:

- Water pills (diuretics)
- Calcium antagonists
- ARBs (Angiotensin receptor blockers)
- Angiotensin Converting Enzyme (ACE) inhibitors
- Beta blockers

In some cases, your doctor may prescribe less common medications, such as…

- Anti-Mineralocorticoids
- Alpha blockers

Nobody will ever expect you to remember these terms, but if your doctor refers to your medications by these names (as they often will) at least you will be able to look them up and find out what they do.

The ways in which these drugs work is usually described by the complicated-sounding names they are given. For instance, calcium antagonists block calcium receptors, diuretics, or water tablets, cause you to pass more urine than usual and a beta blocker blocks beta receptors. How these drugs work will be considered later in this chapter, but for now, commonly used drugs in the commonly used categories will be listed, so you can easily check which sort of drug you are on.

Only the generic names are listed as some older drugs have different trade names depending on which company makes them.

Medication Examples

Drugs will generally work in a similar way if they're in the same category.

The drug companies give names to their particular version of each drug, so each drug will have two names – a generic name which doctors will refer to, and their trade name. In most cases, doctors will use the generic names, though many patients will be more familiar with the trade names.

The packaging of your medications should always display the generic name somewhere, though the trade name will usually be displayed more prominently.

Diuretics

"Thiazide diuretics" is the name given to diuretics in this category. They include…

- Bendroflumethiazide
- Hydrochlorothiazide

Beta-Adrenergic Blocking Agents (Beta Blockers)

If your medication ends in the suffix "-olol", it's a beta blocker. These include…

- Atenolol
- Propranolol
- Metoprolol

Calcium Channel Blocks

Medications ending in the suffix "-dipine" are generally calcium channel blockers:

- Amlodipine
- Isradipine
- Nifedipine

Some calcium channel blockers have different name-types, however:

- Diltiazem
- Verapamil

Angiotensin Converting Enzyme (ACE) Inhibitors

Medications ending in the suffix "-pril" are generally ACE inhibitors:

- Benazepril
- Captopril
- Ramipril
- Perindopril

Angiotensin II Receptor Blockers

Medications ending in the suffix "-artan" are generally ARBs:

- Azilsartan
- Candesartan
- Losartan

What Does My Medication Do?

Medications work to lower blood pressure by:

- Widening your arteries
- Causing more water and sodium to be excreted
- Reducing heart rate

It is perhaps good to consider the analogy of the central heating system here; it takes a higher pressure to pump fluid through narrow pipes than if these pipes were wider. Many of these medications work by relaxing the walls of your arteries, though each drug works in a different way. The pressure needed to pump blood through your arteries falls when the walls of your arteries relax, effectively widening them.

Some medications reduce your heart rate. Some medications also work by encouraging the kidneys to excrete water and sodium, a component of salt. Some medications work by combining some or all of these effects.

Diuretics

These medications work to reduce blood pressure by encouraging your kidneys to excrete sodium into the urine you produce. Diuretic tablets make people urinate more often as water tends to follow sodium into the urine. Your blood pressure is then reduced by the loss of salt and water from your bloodstream.

Beta-Adrenergic Blocking Agents (Beta Blockers)

The walls of your arteries are relaxed by beta blockers, and your heart rate is slowed down.

Calcium Channel Blockers

These medications relax the walls of your arteries to reduce your blood pressure. Some have no major effect on your heart rate, though some can cause it to increase. Your doctor will suggest a calcium channel blocker that doesn't have this effect if they think an increased heart rate will be an issue for you.

Angiotensin Converting Enzyme (ACE) Inhibitors

Certain hormones increase your blood pressure by making your kidneys retain sodium and narrowing your arteries, and ACE inhibitors work to slow down the production of these hormones. ACE inhibitors encourage your kidneys to get rid of sodium and relax the walls of your arteries by stopping these hormones from being produced.

Angiotensin II Receptor Blockers

ARBs encourage sodium excretion in the kidneys and relax artery walls by acting in a similar way to ACE inhibitors.

Which Tablet Is Best?

This is a difficult question to answer. The type of drug you use is much less important than the effectiveness of your treatment, as many scientific studies have found. However, if you are advised to go onto medication, the pragmatic approach is for you and your doctor to find a medication that both treats your hypertension and has no (or tolerable) side effects.

"It is known that lowering blood pressure is beneficial. But there is still a lot of debate about whether any one tablet is better than another, even though many studies have been done to try to answer this question."

Research has shown that some tablets may work better in certain people, but have not found one "best" tablet that works better than the rest. As a result, guidelines exist to advise doctors on which tablets certain people should be given. These guidelines recommend which tablets to try to start with and also what to try if these don't work. All the same, you may have to try a few different medications before you find the one that works for you.

Will I Only Need One Tablet?

Generally speaking, the higher your blood pressure is to start with the more likely you are to need more than one tablet. Some people need to take a combination of tablets, but most get away with just taking one.

Before adding a second tablet, if your blood pressure isn't dangerously high but the first tablet you've tried isn't working, your doctor may suggest swapping you over to a different one.

What Are the Guidelines?

To make sure that the costs of treatment aren't too high and that patients receive the right treatment for them, guidelines have been produced for doctors to follow.

- For patients under the age of 50, ACE inhibitors are the drug of choice
- Diuretics or calcium channel blockers are the drug of choice if you are older than 50 or Afro-Caribbean

The guidelines suggest that you should try combining an ACE inhibitor with either a calcium channel blocker or a diuretic if your first medications don't do the job.

Combining an ACE inhibitor with a calcium blocker and a diuretic is the best option if taking only two medications doesn't work.

	Age 50 and Under	Age 50+ or Afro-Caribbean
1 Tablet	ACE Inhibitor	Diuretic
2 Tablets	ACE inhibitor + Calcium channel blocker OR ACE inhibitor + Diuretic	
3 Tablets	ACE inhibitor + Calcium channel blocker + Diuretic	

Will My Doctor Always Follow These Guidelines?

Evidence suggesting that these combinations work well was used to produce the above guidelines. However, your doctor may have different suggestions that they think will be more appropriate for you, as they know your medical history. If your doctor doesn't strictly follow these guidelines, there's no real cause for concern.

Will I Always Have to Take This Medication?

In most cases, yes. Your blood pressure is likely to return to being high if you stop taking your medication, as hypertension is not something that can usually be cured.

This general rule isn't always true, however. You may be able to stop taking the tablets if you successfully implement lifestyle measures like losing weight or getting more active, this can cause your blood pressure to decrease by itself.

Treating Isolated Systolic Hypertension

Lifestyle modification and in some cases drug treatment is used to treat systolic hypertension, just like any other form of high blood pressure.

Your doctor will try to keep your diastolic blood pressure above 70mmHg if you have to take medications for your systolic hypertension. In those who have isolated systolic hypertension, there is some concern that a diastolic blood pressure below 70mmHg could lead to a heart attack or stroke.

Isolated Diastolic Hypertension Treatments

Whether or not we should treat isolated diastolic hypertension is still under debate amongst doctors. If your diastolic blood pressure is above 90mmHg, the guidelines suggest that doctors should start thinking about offering treatment. That said, especially if you are over 50 years old and have no other risk factors for heart disease, you and your doctor may decide against treating your high diastolic blood pressure if there is no strong evidence to suggest that the treatment is beneficial.

If I Have Hypertension Should I Also Be Taking Treatment for My Cholesterol?

"It used to be thought that if your cholesterol was normal then you did not need to worry about it. It has now been found that if you have had a heart attack or stroke, or suffer from angina, even if your cholesterol is normal then taking treatment to lower it further is beneficial."

If you suffer from a combination of high cholesterol and high blood pressure, your doctor will advise you to take treatments for both as both are risk factors for cardiovascular disease.

Why Has My Doctor Asked Me to Take Medication if My Cholesterol Is Normal?

Some experts believe that it may be beneficial to take medication to lower your cholesterol – even if you have never suffered from a stroke or heart disease and your cholesterol is normal – if you are at high risk of suffering from these conditions in the future.

Whether or not you are advised to take treatment to lower your cholesterol is determined by your cardiovascular risk. There is no such thing as "normal" cholesterol.

There Are Several Different Types of Cholesterol, Are Some Better than Others?

People are often talking about their "total" cholesterol level when they say that their cholesterol is normal. Some cholesterol is beneficial, though, and some is harmful – it isn't just one substance, but a whole group of substances. When your doctor calculates your risk of suffering from future problems related to your high blood pressure they will look at how much "good" and "bad" cholesterol you have.

- HDL cholesterol, or "high-density lipoprotein", is beneficial
- Triglycerides are harmful
- "Low density lipoprotein", or LDL is "bad"

Even if your total cholesterol level is "normal", if you have too much "bad" cholesterol you will be advised to take treatment as your risk of future illness is increased. The pragmatic approach that some doctors and patients take is to try treatment; if it works and has no side effects all well and good, but if it doesn't work or it is not tolerated well the treatment is stopped.

Will Every Doctor Choose to Treat Normal Cholesterol?

The majority of doctors agree that a cholesterol level which is normal should be treated if you have had a stroke, angina or heart attack in the past. That said, if you are at high risk of suffering from these conditions but haven't actually had them yet, not all doctors will agree about whether or not to treat your normal cholesterol. The benefits to be gained by lowering your cholesterol further decrease the lower your cholesterol is to begin with.

Side Effects of Medications and How to Deal with Them

Sadly, side effects are to be expected from all medications that have beneficial effects. This means that they have other effects that may be unrelated to the problem being treated. Tablets apply a broad brush approach, and as a result cause side effects as they have not been designed to target only the exact cause of the problem.

'There is no curing a sick man who believes himself to be in health.'

Henri Amiel, Swiss philosopher.

Does Everyone Suffer from Side Effects?

Most people tolerate blood pressure treatments very well, so it is unlikely that you will have side effects.

Medications are tolerated better by some people when compared to others. Some people seem to be more susceptible to side effects, and this has nothing to do with strength or weakness. If you do experience a side effect with one type of drug, it is possible to swap to a different category which may not give you side effects. When it comes to blood pressure treatments, there are plenty of treatment types to choose from.

Another idea is to change the time that you take your tablet. However, do check with your doctor if this is a good idea for the particular medication you are on.

What Are the Side Effects?

Different side effects are associated with all of the medications in the different treatment categories for hypertension. Usually side effects are nothing to worry about and if they don't bother you too much you can just carry on as normal. The following are the most common side effects, but it is possible to experience something that is not on this list as there are too many possible side effects to list here.

Drug companies are obliged to list all of the potential side effects of a medicine but this doesn't mean that you are likely to suffer from any of these.

- Disorientation
- Changes to kidney function
- Hypokalemia (low potassium level)
- High blood potassium level
- Low blood pressure

Your doctor will run annual blood tests if necessary to keep an eye on your kidney function and potassium levels.

Should I Be Worried about the Length of the List of Side Effects in My Patient Information Leaflet?

Inside the packaging of all medications in the UK, you'll find a "Patient Information Leaflet". Looking through this leaflet is generally a good idea, as people are advised not to take certain medications if they have other pre-existing conditions. That said, unless you are experiencing a side effect and want to know if it's as a result of your medication, it's not really a good idea to worry about the side effects listed. Check the list to make sure you aren't experiencing a second, unrelated ailment, but don't stress yourself into imagining you have symptoms you don't really have.

What Should I Do if I Suffer from a Side Effect?

Talking to your doctor is always a good idea if you notice something wrong after you start taking a medication. Your doctor may want to discuss changing to a different tablet if your side effects are causing real problems. You may also end up sleeping through the worst of the side effects if you take your medication before you go to bed, so changing the time you take your tablets can sometimes be all it takes.

However, some tablets can cause your potassium levels to become too high or too low. Your doctor may need to further investigate the side effects you are experiencing, as on very rare occasions they can be quite serious.

Summing Up

- High blood pressure can be treated with many different types of medication.

- How well your blood pressure responds to its first treatment and how high it was to begin with will determine whether or not you need to take more than one tablet.

- Some people seem to be more susceptible to experiencing side effects than others, but all tablets come with side effects of some sort.

- Your doctor will regularly take blood tests to monitor your potassium levels and kidney function if you are on the sort of tablets that have these side effects.

- If your doctor advises you that your high blood pressure needs treatment it is therefore understandable that you may want to take some time to think about this.

- If you do suffer from a side effect of your medications let your doctor know – they may be able to swap you onto a tablet that suits you better.

- Most people with high blood pressure only need to take one tablet, but unfortunately treatment is usually for life.

- If you need treatment your doctor will advise you on which one is best based on knowledge of any other medical problems you may have, as well as current recommendations.

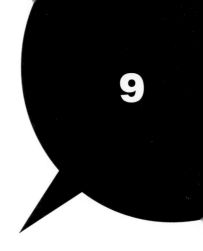

9

Dealing with the Treatment Pros and Cons

For everything in life there are risks as well as benefits and most big decisions that we make are based on balancing these; if it turns out that we think the benefits are greater than the risks we will go ahead. However, with medications, doctors and medical scientists have done the groundwork – they have worked out the benefits and the risks of taking tablets during scientific studies involving large numbers of patients.

Having to take tablets is unappealing to the vast majority of the population. If your blood pressure isn't currently making you feel unwell, it makes sense that you may want some time to consider whether to take a tablet that may give you side effects.

If you try balancing the risks against the benefits, you may find it easier to come to a decision concerning your tablets.

Should I Do What My Doctor Says and Take the Tablets?

Although your doctor is trying to make the best decision for you, you may wish to enter into a more balanced discussion with your doctor about this decision. Your doctor will have come to the conclusion that the benefits of a certain medication will outweigh the risk if they advise you to take it – it's part of their job. You are the one who will have to take the tablets, though, not your doctor.

With this chapter, we hope to arm you with all the information you need to have a balanced, productive conversation with your doctor about the risks and benefits of medication.

> "There are no side effects – only effects. Those we thought of in advance, the ones we like, we call the main, or intended effects, and take credit for them. The ones we didn't anticipate, the ones that came around and bit us in the rear – those are the 'side effects'."
>
> John D. Sterman, Massachusetts Institute of Technology.

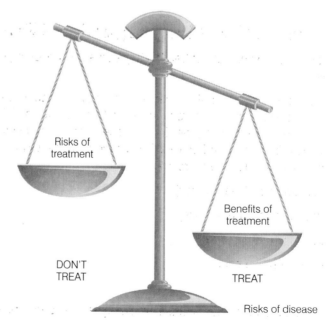

Risks of treatment

Benefits of treatment

DON'T TREAT

TREAT

Risks of disease

Risks vs Benefits

In weighing up risks and benefits of treatment doctors consider:

- The risks that come with the illness
- The risks that come with the medication
- Benefits of treatment

Doctors have to consider the risks of the disease running its course without treatment as well as the risks of treatment. Benefits and risks need to be weighed against each other for every decision that a doctor makes about caring for their patients. How much of a benefit the treatment is likely to have also needs to be taken into consideration, as treatments don't usually fully stop the disease from running its course.

Your doctor will advise that you follow a certain treatment if the medication is beneficial in treating the disease, and they think that the risks of taking this treatment are lower than the risks of letting the disease run its course.

The Risks of Not Treating High Blood Pressure

Chapter Five outlines the risks of not treating hypertension and letting it run its course in greater detail.

To summarise the points made in that chapter, the following issues are more likely to affect you if hypertension runs its course. Therefore treatment for high blood pressure is given with the aim of minimising the risk of these conditions occurring. This does not mean that you will definitely suffer from these conditions if you don't treat your high blood pressure, just that they are more likely.

- Myocardial infarction (heart attack)
- Cerebrovascular accident (stroke)
- CKD (chronic kidney disease)
- Other blood vessel disease
- Angina

Your risk of developing these conditions is even higher if you combine hypertension with high cholesterol and/or diabetes.

Strokes, heart attacks and chest pains are the most common conditions attributed to hypertension. All of these conditions can be disabling or even life threatening and all require treatment, meaning that the stakes in this particular risk benefit calculation are quite high.

Calculating the Risks

How risk is calculated has been covered in detail in Chapter 3. A "cardiovascular risk calculator" is used by doctors to calculate your future risk of suffering from angina, stroke or heart attacks. Your doctor will use the most appropriate risk calculator for your circumstances, as risk can vary depending on which country you live in. Based on this information it gives a percentage risk of you suffering from a heart attack, angina or stroke in the next 10 years.

You can also search for risk calculators on the internet to get a rough idea of your risk. The risk calculator will take into account things like whether or not you have diabetes as well as your sex, cholesterol, blood pressure and age.

What Does This Figure Really Mean?

Put simply, if the risk calculator says you have a 10% risk over the next 10 years, it means you have a 1 in 10 chance of suffering from cardiovascular disease and other adverse consequences of hypertension in the next decade. If you turn this on its head it means that if you don't take treatment for your hypertension you have a 90% (or 9 out of 10) chance of not suffering the adverse consequences of hypertension.

Another way to think about it is this. If ten people who all had a 10% risk (so they all had the same cholesterol, diabetes history, blood pressure, sex and age) were grouped together, in the next 10 years one of the ten people would suffer from angina, stroke or a heart attack.

What Do These Numbers Mean in Terms of Health?

It may seem like only a very small risk if you have a 1 in 10 chance of suffering from the adverse consequences of hypertension. However, the impact that it will have on your life if you are unlucky enough to suffer from angina, a stroke or a heart attack will be massive.

The Benefits of Treating Hypertension

Treating hypertension will not make you feel any better right now. Reducing your risk of suffering from cardiovascular disease in the future is the main benefit of taking treatment for high blood pressure. The greater the reduction in blood pressure, the greater the reduction in risk. A good way of calculating how much your risk has decreased by is to firstly record your calculated risk before treatment and compare this to your risk once your blood pressure has fallen.

How Will Treatment Impact My Cardiovascular Risk?

How much your blood pressure is decreased by treatment will vary from person to person, so it's hard to put an exact number on what your risk will be after treatment. If the treatment only manages to lower your systolic blood pressure by 3mmHg, this will not reduce your risk as much as if it lowers it by 6mmHg.

If you want to figure out how much your risk has been decreased, just use an online risk calculator before you begin treatment and a while after you started taking your medication.

A rough guide is that a blood pressure fall of 5-6mmHg will reduce your risk of a heart attack by around 20%.

It Seems that the Benefits from Treatment Are Large, Are My Calculations Correct?

If you start with a 10% risk of cardiovascular disease in the next ten years reducing this by 20% still leaves you with a risk of 8%. Putting this another way, if your risk of a heart attack in the next 10 years is 1 in 10, taking treatment to reduce this by 20% will still mean your risk is still 0.8 in 10 – which is pretty close to 1 in 10. As good as a 20% reduction in risk may initially seem, it's not quite as large as it sounds.

All of this arithmetic can get a little confusing, but think of it like this:

- 20% of ten is two. So if you reduce your risk of 10% by 20%, you're really just subtracting 2% from your initial risk.

- Ten minus two is eight, so subtracting 2% leaves you with 8%.

So Is the Treatment Worth It if This Number Is So Small?

Most doctors would advise that you do take treatment as they know that the stakes are high and that even a 2% reduction in your risk of suffering from a heart attack is worth trying to achieve. Whether or not you decide treatment is worth it really comes down to how you feel about it. The benefits to be gained from reducing your blood pressure are potentially huge, but you do need to take into account the risks and side effects that come with taking the tablets too.

The Risks of Treatment

Serious side effects are very uncommon in the majority of hypertension treatments. Kidney problems can sometimes occur as a result of taking the tablets, however.

Some people also find that the tablets just make them feel unwell in general, which can be very unpleasant. That said, the majority of people will have no serious side effects from their treatment.

How Do I Decide if the Treatment Is Worth It?

Taking medication to lower your blood pressure will come with a range of benefits and risks, and you will need to work with your doctor to figure these out.

Failing to treat your hypertension will come with risks that need to be considered:

- Heart attacks, angina and strokes are potentially life threatening and require lifelong treatment.
- Your risk of future angina, strokes and heart attacks will be increased if you don't treat your high blood pressure.

Deciding not to treat your hypertension may also have some benefits worth considering:

- You do not currently feel unwell as a result of your high blood pressure.

The benefits of treatment will also need to be considered:

- Your risk of future angina, strokes and heart attacks will be reduced if your hypertension treatment reduces your blood pressure.

… as well as the risks of treatment:

- Your risk will only be reduced by a small amount as a result of this treatment.
- You may feel unwell as a result of your treatment.
- There is a very small risk of serious side effects with treatment.

This All Seems a Bit Overwhelming, Is There a Simple Answer?

Your doctor has had much more experience of calculating the risks and benefits of treatment and will be happy to talk to you about this if you are worried. You don't have to be on your own in deciding whether or not hypertension treatment is right for you.

Whether or not treating your hypertension is the right thing to do does not have a simple answer, unfortunately. That said, it can help to think about it using a pragmatic approach:

- The consequences of high blood pressure can be fatal if left untreated.

- You can keep taking the medication if it seems to be working and isn't causing any side effects.

- You don't have to keep taking the medication if it causes bad side effects and reduces your quality of life.

- So, even though treatment only reduces the risk of these consequences by a small amount it is probably worth trying to take treatment.

Be sure to talk to your doctor if you are taking a medication and decide you want to stop taking it.

Summing Up

- It's really up to you whether you want to take medication or not.

- There are pros and cons of taking tablets, as with everything else in life.

- You may decide to stop taking your medication if it is having a negative effect on your quality of life.

- Most medical practitioners will advise you to take medications to lower your blood pressure as long as they don't give you side effects, or you are able to tolerate the side effects.

- Certainly, reducing the possibility of suffering from a serious consequence of hypertension is worthwhile, but tablets will not reduce this possibility by a large amount.

- Your doctor will offer you sound advice but in the end it is you who will be taking the tablets rather than your doctor.

10

Treating High Blood Pressure without Tablets

Non-prescription medical therapies are often of interest to patients after being diagnosed with hypertension. Some of these therapies may work. Relaxation therapies, herbal medicine and acupuncture are all methods that might be considered. You will need to be objective about the length of time you are going to give this treatment to see if it works.

Patients may find that these therapies do or do not work, but should be aware that while prescription medications have been tested in large trials involving thousands of subjects, herbal remedies do not face this kind of moderation. Hypertension has many potential treatments, but alternative remedies should not be seen as a replacement for medical treatments until they have undergone some more rigorous testing.

Relaxation Therapies

- Short-term hypertension can sometimes be caused by stress
- Long term stress is associated with high blood pressure
- We do not yet know if high blood pressure can be caused by long term stress
- Relaxation techniques may help to lower blood pressure

Things that can lead to cardiovascular disease and increase your blood pressure, such as obesity, drinking, smoking and poor eating habits are all associated with stress – so even if the stress itself doesn't cause high blood pressure, its results can.

This book does not have enough pages to give a thorough review of relaxation therapies. We can, however, give a brief description of the relaxation therapies that have been considered for the treatment of high blood pressure, which include...

- Training yourself to think about your breathing or heartbeat (autogenic training)
- Meditating
- Training yourself to lower your own blood pressure (biofeedback)
- Tai chi
- Progressive muscle relaxation (concentrating on relaxing different muscle groups)
- Guided imagery (focusing on relaxing images)
- Cognitive behavioural therapy (aiming to change the way you think about situations)

Do These Techniques Require Training?

All of these methods are intended for you to be able to do on your own, but there is a learning curve for most of them and you will probably need to be taught the techniques by a certified practitioner. If possible, professional training would be beneficial.

Are Any Methods Better than Others?

The technique that works for you will depend on any number of different personal factors when it comes to relaxation. That said, a number of studies have looked at the use of relaxation techniques in hypertension treatment and identified these as the most widely successful:

- PMR (progressive muscle relaxation)
- CBT (cognitive behavioural therapy)
- Biofeedback

Which Method Is Right for Me?

Trying a few methods and seeing if they have beneficial effects is really the only way of knowing which (if any) technique is right for you. Just make sure you aren't leaving your blood pressure untreated while you try these techniques in the hopes that one will eventually work – it's possible that none of them will.

Chiropractic Manipulation

In recent years, chiropractic has been suggested as a treatment for a range of different conditions. High blood pressure is just one of the many ailments that some chiropractors have suggested their practice can treat. That said, in studies on a large number of patients, chiropractic manipulation on blood pressure has not consistently shown any real benefit.

Herbal Medicines

The distinction between herbal and prescription medicines is often highlighted. However, there is more overlap than is realised. People tend to think of herbal medicines as being collected by botanists, while prescription medicines are produced by chemists in a lab. But many of the medications that doctors prescribe today were originally isolated from fungi and plants.

Herbal remedies that work well against disease are usually incorporated into mainstream medicine, while those that work less well remain as herbal remedies. Fungi, for example, are the source for a number of different treatments for migraine, while digoxin, used to treat abnormal heart rhythms, comes from the foxglove. This movement of successful medications from alternative into mainstream treatment means that mainstream medicines are often tried, tested and more successful than their counterparts that remain under the "herbal" label, though that doesn't mean that herbal remedies have no effect.

Are there Any Herbal Remedies that Treat Hypertension?

It has been suggested that hypertension can be improved by the following herbal remedies. However, there have been no large trials showing convincing evidence that any of these treatments reduce blood pressure.

- Wolf's bane (arnica montana)
- Ignatia
- Cardamom
- Valerian
- Veratrum album
- Natrum muriaticum
- Aurum muriaticum

This list could easily go on much longer. Veratrum album and cardamom are the only two of the above that have scientifically shown some promise for treating high blood pressure. If you do decide to try a herbal remedy for your blood pressure check with your doctor that it is not going to react or interfere with any of your other medications.

Aren't Herbal Medicines Better than Prescribed Medicines if They Don't Have Side Effects?

Some herbal medicines can interact with any prescribed medications that you are on and may have other unwanted effects, though they may not have the same severe side effects as their more tested counterparts.

Should I Avoid Herbal Medications for Treating My Blood Pressure?

This is for you to decide. Whether or not you try herbal medicines is completely up to you. Just be sure to consider the following when you're deciding whether or not you want to try herbal remedies for your hypertension…

- There is good evidence that prescribed medicines reduce blood pressure.
- The effectiveness of herbal remedies in treating hypertension is yet to be proved convincingly.

Can Coenzyme Q10 Improve My Hypertension?

There is some good evidence that Coenzyme Q10 may have a blood pressure lowering effect, but it has not yet been properly compared to conventional medicines for high blood pressure. Most animal and plant cells contain Coenzyme Q10. High blood pressure is just one of a variety of conditions that scientists believe could potentially be treated by it.

Acupuncture

The traditional Chinese medicine 'acupuncture' has been used to treat a wide range of ailments. There have been a few small studies looking at whether acupuncture can lower blood pressure. Acupuncture works on the principle that life energy, or 'qi' flows through specific meridians, or points, and involves the insertion of fine needles into the skin at these points.

So far the jury is out on acupuncture. Some studies of acupuncture have found it to be ineffective, while others have suggested it could be beneficial. The problem is that just because a therapy has worked well for one person, it does not mean that it will work well in everybody.

"Acupuncture is used in many NHS general practices, as well as the majority of hospices and pain clinics in the UK."

Is There Anything to Be Said about Alternative Treatments?

Especially if they have found one that has worked particularly well for them, many patients are willing to swear by the effectiveness of alternative treatments. Some people's blood pressure may even fall for a reason completely unrelated to the therapy, so they will support that therapy without it having helped at all.

How Do Doctors Test to See if Medicines Work?

Doctors will compare a medicine against a placebo (or sugar pill) in many people if they think it may be beneficial. If there are already therapies that are known to be good at treating diseases any new therapy has to be tested against the best treatments that are already available.

The medicine has to prove more effective than the placebo in a significant number of these people before the doctor will say that the treatment works. In order to find its way into mainstream medicine, the new treatment also needs to prove to be as good as, or better than, other existing treatments.

Is This How Alternative Treatments Are Tested?

Small numbers of patients are often used when trialling alternative treatments against placebos. In most of these trials, the alternative treatments haven't shown any real benefit. Further investigation is being carried out into the few treatments that have shown promise, such as Coenzyme Q10.

The Risks of Alternative Treatments

Taking prescribed medications that are well known to treat high blood pressure is the most sensible thing to do if your blood pressure is dangerously high.

Provided you continue meeting with your doctor to check results, there is usually no harm in taking alternative treatments. Your doctor will recommend that you switch to a prescribed medication if the alternative treatment is not improving your blood pressure.

"The main risk of taking an alternative treatment is that you will not seek medical help and take a medication that is known to be beneficial when you really need to."

Summing Up

- Hypertension has many different promoted alternative remedies. There is no evidence to say that most of these work, as they have not been scientifically studied. Some alternative remedies have been scientifically studied, but have shown no real positive results. Some have shown promise, however, including Coenzyme Q10, acupuncture and relaxation remedies.

- Provided you are willing to take prescribed medications if the alternative remedies don't work, most doctors will have no problem with you trying alternative therapies if your blood pressure is only mildly elevated.

- If you have moderate or severely high blood pressure then most doctors would recommend that you take a prescribed treatment for this.

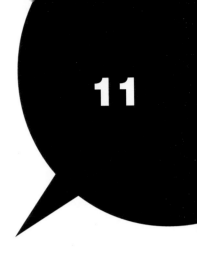

11

Planning Your Blood Pressure Treatment

Before you can change your lifestyle, you need the power of knowledge. There have been many suggestions throughout this book about how to combat high blood pressure. By now, you should have a stronger understanding of blood pressure, and why it is important that you treat your high blood pressure or keep your normal blood pressure in the healthy range.

If you do have hypertension, there are things you can do to improve your future health. If you have a young family it is ideal to get them involved in your plan because if they can get used to a healthy lifestyle they are less likely to suffer from hypertension later in life. You can protect yourself against cardiovascular disease by reducing your blood pressure by even a small amount, and an action plan may even be able to reduce your blood pressure to normal.

As hypertension is just one factor that contributes to heart attacks, angina and strokes, your personal plan to tackle hypertension should also take into account other risk factors for these diseases. In this chapter, we will help you create your own personal plan for tackling high blood pressure by bringing all of your options together in one place.

Be sure to include things like giving up smoking and eating a healthier diet in your action plan, as these are vital for your overall health. It can also be helpful to get your family on board in the planning of your action plan, as they can suggest healthy activities that you can all do together.

An Exercise Program

Your risk of suffering from strokes, heart attacks and angina will be reduced if you take up regular exercise, and this will also lower your blood pressure. Doing regular exercise will also help you to sleep well and combat stress.

Often the monotony of having done the same thing all day can cause mental fatigue that permeates the whole of your body and leaves you wanting to do no more than sit on the sofa. We tend to feel exhausted at the end of the day, whether we've been at school or work, or even if we're retired.

A good exercise program can actually make you feel more awake and energetic, whether you believe it or not (though you will have to get used to the exercise first!)

You will function and feel so much better if you're able to devote 20 to 30 minutes to exercise each day.

Planning Your Workout Routine

1   Log out of Facebook or turn off the TV – get rid of your distractions for now.

2   Give some thought to the types of activities you'd enjoy, or which exercises you think you could enjoy if you gave them a chance. You may have to think back to the exercises you enjoyed when you were younger if it's been a while.

3   Consider your friends: Do they exercise? Could you join them, or convince them to join you if they aren't already active? The whole process will be more fun if you're able to get together as a group, and you'll find it much easier to stay motivated.

4 Join a club. If you don't think you will have the motivation to exercise by yourself and can't persuade your friends to join you, think about joining a club. The sort of clubs that are useful are not gyms, but clubs where you have to interact with other people and your presence is missed if you don't turn up. For example, a badminton club, or running group.

5 If you have children, think about whether it is possible to get them to exercise with you. But remember that young children will not be able to exercise as vigorously as you, so you may need to incorporate them into just small parts of your exercise routine.

6 Get a piece of paper and a pen and write your plan down.

7 Choose a date (not too far away!) and write it down on your plan. You may be more likely to stick to your plan if you write down when you're going to exercise and how long. Leave it somewhere you and your family can all see it to hold yourself accountable.

8 Keep a record. In a spreadsheet or exercise diary, write down what you did and for how long every time you exercise. Writing down how you feel after each session can also be helpful. This will help you to see if you've started skipping sessions, but will also allow you to get a better idea of how you're improving.

9 Don't give up. The first couple of weeks of any exercise program are the hardest, but if you can persevere it will get easier.

10 Build up gradually. Underneath the date you are going to start write down subsequent dates that you are going to exercise on. Make sure to build up the time that you exercise gradually - over a couple of weeks or so.

Changing Your Diet

In a time-pressured society it is all too easy to eat on the hoof and not think too much about what you are actually eating. But if you want to reduce your high blood pressure, eating less salt and losing a bit of weight (if you're overweight) can be a good step. Also, if you have children, getting them to think that healthy eating is normal will be of huge benefit to them later in life.

There are also ways other than lowering your blood pressure that dietary measures like cutting down on sugary or fatty foods and eating more vegetables and fruits can lower your risk of cardiovascular disease. As well as specifically trying to tackle your blood pressure, it's a good idea to change what you eat in a way that will promote the general fitness of your arteries and heart.

It's really important that you try to start eating healthily if you're at all worried about your blood pressure.

Dropping the Pounds

If you are overweight, for the sake of your health, you should think about losing a few pounds. A small reduction in food at meal times, combined with cutting out snacks between meals, is a sustainable approach that won't leave you ravenous. You're at a higher risk of a range of illnesses if you're overweight, including…

- High blood pressure
- Heart disease and strokes
- Diabetes

Am I Overweight because of a Slow Metabolism?

As a general rule, no. If you are overweight it means that you eat too much for you and you need to cut down on the amount you eat. People who are of an ideal weight will often have a slower metabolism than those who are overweight.

I Have Tried Many Diets but They Never Work

Some diets advertise truly miraculous results, and there are so many different diets to choose from. Gradually cutting down the amount that you eat, however, is often the best approach. Fad diets may sound flashy, but they rarely work as well as simply cutting out the snacks and making your portion sizes a little smaller. Even if you are not overweight a change in your diet to include more healthy types of food can be very beneficial.

Can I Lose Weight through Exercise?

Exercise on its own is not as effective in weight loss as a healthy diet. That said, once you've lost the weight, exercise will help you to keep it off. Starting to exercise and eat less at the same time is the best way to go.

Changing the Food that You Eat

You can help protect yourself against strokes and heart disease by eating a healthy diet rich in vegetables and fruit, and improve your blood pressure by eating less salt. We discussed this in Chapter Seven.

It may be a good idea to check out the DASH diet (**www.dashdiet.org**), which has many low-salt, healthy eating recipes. But even with a normal cookbook, it's easy to identify the recipes that don't call for lots of salt or fat, and that are full of fruit and vegetables.

Changing Your Diet

Every day for two or three days, record everything that you normally eat. Keep this record so you can look at it later on.

Look at this list and work out where you can swap an unhealthy for a healthy option, for example a chocolate bar for a fruit bar, or a bag of chips for a baked potato.

Reduce the amount of salt you add to your food gradually (over a few weeks).

Try not to buy too many ready prepared meals, or if you do buy these meals check to see that they are low salt, healthy options.

Make a plan to eat at least five portions of vegetables or fruit every day. This may sound like a lot, but a glass of juice in the morning will already have given you one portion! Take note of how you are going to get all of your portions.

Pick a few evenings in the week where you and your family can cook and eat a healthy recipe together.

At the beginning or end of each month, write down everything you eat for another few days and compare this to the original list. This will allow you to see where you have improved, but also how you can eat healthier the following month.

Should I Take Antioxidant Vitamins?

The best way to make sure that you take in the right amount of vitamins is to eat a healthy and balanced diet. A lot of people think that a healthy diet should include antioxidant vitamin supplements. Although these substances are beneficial when they are contained in vegetables, scientific studies have shown that they lose their benefit when they are taken as pills.

Sadly, there isn't actually any evidence which would suggest that they're much use at all. It could actually be the case that taking antioxidants in the form of vitamin pills is actively bad for you.

Drinking Less Alcohol

The Department of Health's guidelines concerning how much alcohol we can safely drink were changed in 2016, taking into consideration the better understanding we now have of how regular drinking can increase cancer risk. For most people, sticking to the daily recommended amount is not going to cause them any harm. Most of us are familiar enough with the old guideline of 21 units for women and 28 units for men, but the new guidelines are as follows:

- Both women and men are advised to limit their intake to 14 units or less each week.

- Consider cutting down by having a few alcohol-free days every week.

- Spread your drinking over 3 or more days if you regularly drink as much as 14 units a week.

A wide range of medical conditions can result from excessive amounts of alcohol, such as hypertension, stomach ulcers and liver disease. Hypertension and other future health problems may become an issue if you regularly drink more than the recommended weekly amount.

"And the day came when the risk to remain tight in a bud was more painful than the risk it took to blossom."

Anais Nin, writer.

Stopping Smoking

Smoking is an addiction and it is very easy to keep finding excuses not to give up this habit. You will always find a reason to delay quitting so you need to make a date to stop and stick to it – no excuses. Stopping smoking has been covered in detail in Chapter 7.

Smokers are at a much higher risk of suffering from strokes or heart disease, though smoking doesn't directly cause high blood pressure. As part of your general aim to reduce cardiovascular risk, any action plan to tackle hypertension should ideally include a plan to stop smoking.

Be successful in changing one thing before moving on to another. Your personal plan for tackling hypertension will need to include a feasible plan for giving up smoking, as it's something that's generally very difficult to do. This needs to be a plan that doesn't allow for excuses like "I'll give up smoking after the weekend", "I'll just smoke socially" or "after the kids have started back to school."

Write the date that you are going to stop on a piece of paper in big letters, sign it and put it where your family can see it. It could help if you draw up some sort of agreement or contract with your partner, friends or kids.

Some people like to turn over a new leaf all at once. Remember to choose carefully when you're going to incorporate quitting into your plan. You may find your action plan too difficult to cope with if you try to make too many changes at once, and quitting smoking may be the last straw.

Your doctor might suggest that you should give up smoking as the first part of your plan, as it's such a huge risk factor for strokes and heart disease. Just remember to put the other parts of your personal plan into action once you've given up smoking – you won't be done after one change, unfortunately!

Tips for Giving Up

The following are just some pointers to refresh your memory. For more information on giving up smoking, read Chapter Seven.

- Remind yourself of why you're quitting
- If you have friends who also want to quit, do it together
- Look into nicotine gums and patches, as these can make it easier
- Ask your GP for advice
- Keep away from situations in which you would normally smoke
- Pick a date and stick to it

A Partnership with Your Doctor

Your doctor will be delighted if you are taking an active part in taking care of yourself, but don't forget that your doctor is a valuable source of information. Keeping your blood pressure low should be something for both you and your doctor to aim for. But don't forget, while you will probably be impatient to see your blood pressure fall, your doctor will know that these things take time.

Keeping you healthy and well is your doctor's job. But it should also be your priority. If you want to improve your health, the best way to do it is to form a strong partnership with your doctor. The best way to make sure you stay healthy and happy is to combine your effort with the knowledge of your doctor.

Mention to your GP that you want to take an active part in trying to lower your blood pressure, if you have hypertension.

- Get them to tell you about healthy eating and weight loss
- Ask for advice about giving up smoking
- Ask them about whether your alcohol intake should be reduced
- Ask them about recommended exercise programs for you

To help you achieve your goals, your GP may even be able to signpost you to some local groups or clubs.

Trust your doctor's advice, and try not to get frustrated if you have setbacks or if you aren't making progress as quickly as you thought you would.

Summing Up

- How your health develops is very much down to you.

- Your risk of having to take tablets for hypertension can be reduced if you put the suggestions into action right now, before your blood pressure becomes elevated. You can also help your children to avoid suffering from hypertension in their later lives if you get them involved in your plan today.

- The tips in this chapter will help to keep your blood vessels and heart healthy, as well as potentially lowering your blood pressure.

- If you ask your doctor for advice and let them know you want to take an active role in improving your blood pressure, they will be happy to help.

- Don't forget, your doctor is there to help.

- If you already have hypertension, it is not too late to start your plan.

- Doctors can give you tablets to treat your blood pressure, but it is much better if by developing your own personal plan to tackle hypertension your blood doesn't become elevated in the first place.

Help List

General Information

Blood Pressure Information Resource
www.bpassoc.org.uk
Email: info@bpassoc.org.uk
The UK's leading resource on high blood pressure or hypertension.

British and Irish Hypertension Society
www.bihsoc.org
Address: Jackie Howarth, BIHS Executive Assistant, On Call Suite, Glenfield Hospital, Groby Road, Leicester LE3 9QP.
Tel: 0116 250 2605.
Email: bihs@le.ac.uk
A forum for professionals working in the field of hypertension and cardiovascular disease in the UK and Ireland.

High Blood Pressure Foundation
www.hbpf.org.uk
Address: Dept of Medicinal Sciences, Western General Hospital, Edinburgh EH4 2XU.
Tel: 0131 332 9211.
For general information and patient support.

Your GP Surgery
Your local GP and practice nurse will be very happy to give you advice or point you in the direction of a local support group for any of the issues covered in this book.

Giving Up Smoking

Smokefree
www.nhs.uk/smokefree
Tel: 0300 123 1044
The NHS online resource for people who want to quit smoking. Smokefree offers free advice and support, and an option to call or message an expert for more information.

Diet Advice

The Mediterranean and DASH Diets for Healthy Weight Loss, Lower Blood Pressure & Cholesterol

www.dashdiet.org

Dietary Approaches to Stop Hypertension, or TASH, was developed to lower blood pressure without medication in research sponsored by the US National Institutes of Health.

Patient UK

www.patient.co.uk

For general advice on health and medical conditions. Use the search box to find advice on healthy eating and weight loss.

Exercise Advice

The Keep Fit Association

www.keepfit.org.uk/
Tel: 01403 266000
Email: kfa@emdp.org
Brings people in similar areas together to exercise.

Patient

www.patient.info
Tel: +4420 3751 0486
Email: clinicalcontent@patient.info
Patient empowers everyone to take charge of their health. They help people feel better and live longer by providing trusted clinical information, written and reviewed by an extensive network of doctors and healthcare professionals.

Walking & Hiking Information

www.whi.org.uk
Email: contactus@whi.org.uk
A website with information about getting involved in walking and hiking, and ideas for places to go for the best walks.

Alternative Therapies

The Complementary and Natural Healthcare Council
www.cnhc.org.uk
Address: 83 Victoria Street, LONDON SW1H 0HW.
Tel: 0203 178 2199.
Email: info@cnhc.org.uk.
For information on complementary healthcare providers.

General Hypnotherapy Standards Council & General Hypnotherapy Register
www.general-hypnotherapy-register.com
Address: GHSC & GHR, PO BOX 204, Lymington S)41 6WP.
Email: admin@general-hypnotherapy-register.com
The General Hypnotherapy Standards Council (GHSC) and the General Hypnotherapy Register (GHR) are the UK's largest and most prominent organisations within the field of hypnotherapy and together present an exemplary model for the simultaneous protection of the public and the provision of practitioner credibility services.

Sources

Acupuncture - NHS – **https://www.nhs.uk/conditions/acupuncture**

Alcohol units - NHS – **https://www.nhs.uk/live-well/alcohol-support/calculating-alcohol-units**

Anaemia - Irishhealth.com - **http://www.irishhealth.com/article.html?con=593**

Blood pressure lowering, fibrinolysis enhancing and antioxidant activities of cardamom (Elettaria cardamomum). – PubMed – NCBI – **https://www.ncbi.nlm.nih.gov/pubmed/20361714**

Causes of fainting - HSE.ie - **https://www.hse.ie/eng/health/az/f/fainting/causes-of-fainting-.html**

Dehydration - Symptoms and causes - Mayo Clinic - **https://www.mayoclinic.org/diseases-conditions/dehydration/symptoms-causes/syc-20354086**

Health Matters: combating high blood pressure – GOV.UK – **https://www.gov.uk/government/publications/health-matters-combating-high-blood-pressure/health-matters-combating-high-blood-pressure**

Health Risks of Being Overweight | NIDDK – **https://www.niddk.nih.gov/health-information/weight-management/health-risks-overweight**

The Mediterranean and DASH Diets for Healthy Weight Loss, Lower Blood Pressure & Cholesterol – **https://www.dashdiet.org**

Obesity | The Nuffield Trust – **https://www.nuffieldtrust.org.uk/resource/obesity**

Relaxation techniques: Try these steps to reduce stress – Mayo Clinic – **https://www.mayoclinic.org/healthy-lifestyle/stress-management/in-depth/relaxation-technique/art-20045368**

Statistics on Obesity, Physical Activity and Diet, England, 2019 – NHS Digital – **https://digital.nhs.uk/data-and-information/publications/statistical/statistics-on-obesity-physical-activity-and-diet/statistics-on-obesity-physical-activity-and-diet-england-2019**

Turning the tide on tobacco: Smoking in England hits a new low – Public health matters – **https://publichealthmatters.blog.gov.uk/2018/07/03/turning-the-tide-on-tobacco-smoking-in-england-hits-a-new-low**